in the hands of every person truly seeking to become advocates for their own health and wellness. Reading it will inspire, educate and empower us all."

—**Rachel Gerrol**, *Co-Founder & CEO, NEXUS*

"I've watched Dr. Gedroic work her magic with some of my closest friends. She has a unique approach to healing and staying healthy. If you're interested in your health, her book is a must-read!"

—**Danny Wegman**, *Chairman, Wegman's Food Markets*

"I love every word of *A Nation of Unwell*. Dr. Gedroic cogently explains why taking care of our insides like we do our outsides is the path to alleviating the suffering brought on by chronic disease. Understanding how the gut microbiome, liver, and gallbladder work to nourish and detoxify us is something we all should have been taught but most weren't. Following her clear, step-by-step nutrition and self-care plan is a prescription for feeling vibrantly well in body, energy, and mood while preventing and reversing chronic conditions—without relying on the long-term use of prescription medications. We can do this ourselves, and Dr. Gedroic shows us why and how to do it."

—**Nancy Weiser, MBA**, *Certified Health Coach, Founder Weiser Choices*

Advance Praise for *A Nation of Unwell*

"If you want to understand and know why people get sick and the road to healing and recovery this is the book to read. Dr Kristine Gedroic has done a great service to all of us by clearly defining the common origins of modern chronic illnesses and their cures. This book contains the most comprehensive summary of the connection between genes, epigenetic activity, microbiome, neuroplasticity, metabolic activity, inflammation, and more. I recommend it to all who are interested in preventing illness but also finding common solutions to their reversal and return to total well-being. I will use it myself as a guide and suggest it as a must read for patients, health care providers, medical students, and anyone who wants to understand the scientific basis of the emerging paradigm for health at all levels of experience: physical emotional, societal, and spiritual."

—*Deepak Chopra, MD, FACP, co-founder of the Chopra Center for Wellbeing, founder of the Chopra Foundation, world-renowned pioneer in integrative medicine and personal transformation, and author of numerous books including* You Are the Universe *and* Quantum Healing

"A groundbreaking book, *A Nation of Unwell* offers a new roadmap for healing. Dr. Gedroic explains why the body succumbs to disease and exactly what needs to be done to restore balance and health. I recommend it as a must-read for anyone who wants to live a life of wellness."

—*Andrew Weil, MD, founder and director of the Arizona Center for Integrative Medicine at the University of Arizona, founder and chairman of The Weil Foundation, world-renowned leader and pioneer in the field of integrative medicine, and author of numerous books including* Mind Over Meds *and* Fast Food, Good Food

"Dr. Gedroic offers thoughtful explanations and game plans for chronically unwell people who should be thriving in life rather than desperately coping with symptoms."

—*Mehmet Oz, MD, attending physician, New York Presbyterian/Columbia University, host of* The Dr. Oz Show, *and co-author of numerous books including* Food Can Fix It

"As Americans continue to suffer from chronic illness, inflammation, and stress at alarmingly increasing rates, this book provides an inspiring tool for patients to reclaim their health and begin to understand the potential underlying causes of their conditions, so that they can start on the road to feeling well."

—**Ray Chambers,** *World Health Organization Ambassador for Global Strategy*

"Dr. Gedroic has written the go-to book for patients and their families who are suffering from chronic illness and don't know what to do. It provides a clear understanding of not only <u>why</u> they are sick but also provides a roadmap of what they can <u>do</u> to get better. *A Nation of Unwell* provides a comprehensive overview of our dysfunctional medical system and all of the areas that need to be addressed to allow the body to heal. This book is a must-read for those who are ready to embrace their journey towards healing, and for those who wish to be proactive in not allowing their bodies to become ill."

—**Neil Nathan, MD**, *author of* Toxic, Heal Your Body

"All humans have one thing in common ... we want to FEEL good. Dr. Gedroic has written a must-read debut book for anyone looking to achieve optimal wellness. Her clear and detailed explanations of why we have become a nation of unwell offers readers a fresh perspective on how they can take steps to reclaim their health and discover the root causes of their ailments."

—**Jesse Itzler**, *entrepreneur, New York Times bestselling author of* Living with a SEAL *and an owner of the Atlanta Hawks*

"I came to Dr. Gedroic as a patient after being told by experts at several leading research hospitals that there were no treatment options available to me until the symptoms of my diagnosis became more severe. Dr. Gedroic not only identified the root causes of my condition, but she offered a course of treatment to address these underlying issues that gave me hope and, more importantly, a pathway to complete recovery and health. This book belongs

A
NATION
of
UNWELL

···························

WHAT'S GONE WRONG?

KRISTINE L. GEDROIC, MD
with Valerie A. Latona

Published by LCR Publishing

LCR

ISBN 978-1-7324446-0-7 (hardcover)
ISBN 978-1-7324446-1-4 (paperback)
ISBN 978-1-7324446-2-1 (ebook)

Cover Design: Fresh Design
Interior Design: GKS Creative, Nashville
Illustrations © Robert Margulies

This book may be purchased for educational, business, or sales promotional use. For information, please call 973-993-4445, X411.

The information in this book is designed to help the reader make informed decisions about his/her health. It is not intended as a medical prescription or to replace the advice of the reader's own physician or other medical professional. It is not intended to replace any medical treatment offered by the reader's own doctor(s). Every reader should consult a medical professional in matters relating to health, especially if you have preexisting medical conditions. The author(s) and publisher do not accept responsibility for any adverse effects individuals may claim to experience, whether directly or indirectly, from the information contained in this book. The names and identifying characteristics of patients have been changed to protect their privacy.

Publisher's Cataloging-In-Publication Data
(Prepared by The Donohue Group, Inc.)

Names: Gedroic, Kristine L., author. | Latona, Valerie A., author.
Title: A nation of unwell : what's gone wrong? / Kristine L. Gedroic, MD, with Valerie A. Latona.
Description: Morristown, NJ : LCR Publishing, [2019] | Includes bibliographical references and index.
Identifiers: ISBN 9781732444607 (hardcover) | ISBN 9781732444614 (paperback) | ISBN 9781732444621 (ebook)
Subjects: LCSH: Self-care, Health. | Chronic diseases--Prevention. | Medicine, Preventive. | Diet therapy.
Classification: LCC RA776.95 .G44 2019 (print) | LCC RA776.95 (ebook) | DDC 613--dc23

This book is dedicated to my grandmother,
Mary Elizabeth Bemish Wegman.
Your light still shines on.
Thank you for helping me to see the way.

CONTENTS

A Letter from Lauren

Dr. Gedroic,

During the first drive to your office, I tried desperately to put the recurring negative thoughts out of my mind that you would be like every other medical professional I'd seen, glazing over my symptoms and quickly prescribing a strong medication without hesitation. Part of me knew that somehow this wouldn't be the case, but I couldn't completely deny the deep fear inside me.

As a little girl, I aspired to be a physician, as they were the true superheroes to me, coming in and "saving the day" by figuring out the mysterious cause of someone's migraine or the obscure rash sprawling across one's leg. That is, until I became sick. It is then that I realized that so many physicians would rather push medications than spend time to find the root cause of an issue like mine.

I still remember the first words you ever said to me: "Wow, you have quite the story." This was the first time a doctor recognized what I had gone through, acknowledged it, and validated it. It was then that I knew I was in good hands. After I left that first appointment, I cried with relief because, for the first time in two years, I knew I would survive.

I clearly remember the day I started to turn the corner. Walking past a box of my school papers, I noticed a sticker I bought when I toured Stanford University. I thought that if I could come out of this process whole and stronger than I had been going into it, I surely could attend Stanford. It was the first time in almost six months I thought again about college and the future.

I now have only my final exams left before I am officially done with high school. Less than four months ago, given the state of my health, I questioned whether or not I'd finish in time to prepare for AP exams and graduate. And yet, here I am cured, free from a lifetime of medications—and feeling, finally, like my old self.

Words cannot convey the gratitude I have for all that you have done for me. You are a true doctor and what all doctors should strive to be. Not only have you restored my health, but you have also helped restore my faith in myself by helping me to understand that I can and will do whatever I set my mind to. I had lost my way and couldn't see beyond my illness and the darkness that consumed me, but you became my white light.

Thank you for finding the root cause of my sickness and for not just prescribing more pills. Thank you for listening to me. Thank you for being my superhero.

Thank you for everything.

Lauren K.

Introduction

Every day, patients come to my clinic, The Gedroic Medical Institute in Morristown, New Jersey, and ask, "What is wrong with me?" In most cases, they've already seen numerous doctors, received multiple diagnoses, and are taking prescription medications—and still don't feel well. Others have received no official diagnosis but remain unwell and are unwilling to accept a life of feeling sick and having to take prescription medicines with myriad side effects. The most common conditions patients seek my help about include chronic fatigue syndrome, autoimmune disease, fibromyalgia, irritable bowel syndrome (IBS), gastroesophageal reflux disease (GERD), and attention deficit hyperactivity disorder (ADHD), as well as many more. Patients come to my clinic not to receive another "label" but, instead, to finally get well.

But what do these disease labels really mean, particularly if a patient still isn't feeling well after receiving a diagnosis? And what do these disease labels mean to the almost 117 million Americans who are coping with chronic health problems? In order to understand the answer, we must look deeper at what is happening with our health and in medicine today to answer the question: *Why are we so sick?*

To put it quite bluntly, something is terribly wrong or chronic disease wouldn't be on a consistent upward trajectory. This should come as no great surprise to the millions of people who are chronically unwell, who are struggling for answers, and who are desperate for a return to some semblance of normalcy in their lives. Despite rapid and impressive advances in medicine today, the average American is sicker than ever, depending on more than one prescription medication just to have a day without symptoms but never fully feeling well. They're coping every day with chronic pain, digestive upset, behavioral disorders, and more that are affecting their quality of life.

So why is our health failing us? And why do so many people now see it as almost inevitable, at some point in their lives, to be diagnosed with chronic illnesses like digestive disorders, autoimmune diseases, and cancer?

What's also considered inevitable: the drugs we're prescribed to help us live with these illnesses, to cope with our symptoms, and to extend our lifespan. Having learned to accept needing medication to stay well, we think nothing of taking not merely one, but two, three, four, or sometimes even five medications daily without stopping to ask, *Why should I need all this?* And we think nothing of having to take a drug every day for the rest of our lives. This is *not* normal and should not be normal. At no point are we taking the time to ask the question of *why* we're getting these diseases at a rapidly escalating rate and, most importantly, what's underlying these diseases and triggering them in the first place.

What this means is that we're living our lives on 50 percent power or even less. We have become numb to the fact that this is not okay, this is not how our bodies should be feeling, and this is not how our bodies should be working. And countless children are also unhealthy today. Why are our children unwell? This loudly brings to the fore the question *What is really going wrong?*

Just recently, I was talking with one of the top New York pediatric neurologists and we both agreed: *Kids are not healthy today.* Kids are sicker, with more diagnoses of a variety of conditions, than ever before. And their waistlines are growing, too, with more and more kids being diagnosed as overweight and even obese. The latest statistics estimate that one in four children, or fifteen to eighteen million children aged seventeen and younger, now suffer from a chronic health problem.[1] These statistics are absolutely staggering and must change if we are to ensure the health of generations to come.

A Different Way of Looking at Disease

Health today is being viewed in *two* dimensions, which is why things are going wrong. Let's walk through one of my patient visits and shine a light on how one might see health and wellness in *three* dimensions, which is how it needs to be viewed in order for patients to be able to recover optimal wellness.

Rachel comes to my clinic after having seen a multitude of doctors. She's been told she has chronic fatigue syndrome (which is the reason she has no energy); she has insomnia (which is why she doesn't sleep well); she has irritable bowel syndrome (which explains why she's frequently bloated and gassy); she has migraines (which is the reason she has frequent headaches); and she has depression (which explains why she is feeling sad about life and doesn't want to participate in her normal daily activities anymore). Depression is a common "tag-on" condition that many chronically ill people are diagnosed with for good reason. When you're unable to enjoy your life because you're not feeling well on a daily basis, it's easy to feel sad and hopeless about pretty much everything. But it goes even deeper than that: what is going on in our bodies directly affects our brains. When the body is out of balance, the mind typically is too. This explains why depression rates, which mirror our rising overall disease rates, are at an all-time high. At the latest count, sixteen million Americans are affected, with one-third not responding to medical treatments.[2]

Including depression, Rachel now has five labels as to why she's not feeling well and has been given five different prescription drugs to treat each of these "conditions," with each of the drugs coming with its own litany of side effects. Five drugs for five conditions. If Rachel takes all the medication prescribed, she hopes she will feel better, but there's no guarantee.

But what do these diagnoses really mean? In other words, *what is really going on with Rachel?*

What's alarming is that the average adult today is not that different from Rachel. The majority of Americans simply accept that they will require medication to stay well at some point in their lives. What's worse is that we're now accepting that our children require medication in order to stay well.

Let's go deeper to examine the issue. We must first accept that we have no definition for "optimal wellness" in medicine today. In other words, medicine is not operating with a "maintain wellness" model; instead, we are operating with an "acute care" model, which means we use medication to control symptoms. Today, a patient is "well" simply when they feel well and have no disease diagnoses. How then can we explain it when that very same patient, who perceives themselves to be "well" one day, is diagnosed with cancer, an autoimmune disease, or a neurological condition the next month or year? How does this happen? It didn't simply occur in one day, one month, or even one year. It represents a growing problem in the body that often has taken *years* to develop. Why, then, is our present model not catching these conditions early on, before we have a real problem to deal with? Simply put, we need to improve how we are approaching and dealing with symptoms and disease.

The "why" or reason we aren't catching conditions before they become evident has to do with the fact that medicine today is practiced as a linear model. "Rachel, you have Symptom X, therefore you have Condition Y and must take Medication Z to feel better." This tells us nothing about how Condition Y developed in the first place.

The clues as to how Condition Y developed are Rachel's symptoms, her body's only way of communicating to her that something's just not right in its effort to get well. Our bodies cannot verbally say, "I am out of balance" or "I am dehydrated." Instead, we might get a headache. Once we start to understand that symptoms are powerful clues as to what's wrong with the body's underlying process, we can start to unravel the mystery of how we get sick.

I often liken health to a seesaw. When balanced, we feel well. When out of balance, we don't feel well, symptoms manifest themselves and, if continually ignored, disease sets in. In fact, most disease today means "too much of something that shouldn't be there," or a stress on the system (e.g., a toxin or an infection), or "too little of something that should be there," or a lack of key balancers (e.g., essential nutrients the cells need to stay healthy). Once health begins being viewed in these dynamic three-dimensional terms and healing is directed at "balancing out the seesaw again," one can see how true recovery might be possible.

Identifying the Clues or Symptoms

To understand the potential imbalances in Rachel's body, we started our meeting by talking about her health history for more than an hour. We actually began not with her but with her family. The questions included: How healthy were your parents, and what was your home environment like when you were growing up? Were you born via vaginal delivery or C-section? Did you drink formula or were you breastfed? What was your early infancy and childhood health like? What kinds of foods did you eat while you were growing up? These types of questions helped me start to identify whether there were enough balancers or nutrients in her system from the very beginning, laying the foundation for health or eventual illness.

Other questions we discussed pertained to stressors on her system: When did her symptoms develop, how did they evolve, and in what order? What was her living environment at different times in her life? Has there been any known exposure to mold, insect bites, pets, or anything that could have added to why she feels unwell, including any foreign travel, hobbies like painting and gardening, or exposure to chemicals in the home or in her environment? We explored everything together in an effort to identify when and how the symptoms began.

Rachel's symptoms are my clues along the way. They tell me a great deal about the ultimate diagnosis. In fact, they often weave a beautiful web of truth around how a patient like Rachel got sick in the first place and exactly what must be done to unravel the illness.

As doctors, instead of blunting symptoms with medication, we must start to interpret them to correct the underlying health issues. I often use a smoke detector analogy with my patients: If a smoke detector unexpectedly went off in your home, would you first try to determine whether there was a fire or would you dismantle the detector? You would obviously look for, and put out, the fire first. Yet most medication dismantles the detector (i.e., the symptoms), and doctors are not being trained to look for the fire (i.e., the underlying cause of the symptoms). But medicine can and should put out the fire first. This book begins the conversation about how to do just this.

Sometimes it's merely one thing that's wrong. A patient, adult or child, might have an undiagnosed virus or bacterial infection that his/her body can't fight off. He/she may be getting exposed to one particular toxin or too many toxins in very high levels. And in some cases, a patient may have nutritional deficiencies: she may lack simple amino acids, minerals, or specific vitamins to maintain wellness. This is surprisingly quite common with many adults and children today, despite believing their diets to be adequate. But most of the time, it is numerous undiagnosed cellular issues that have added up over the years in that patient to trigger their disease or are the reason they feel unwell.

In Rachel's case, we needed to identify the multitude of stressors on her system, including toxins and infections, along with the needed balancers to restore health. As it turns out, Rachel had an undiagnosed bacterial infection, viral infections, and exposure to certain toxins that were at the root of her problems. Once those stressors were resolved and her system was rebalanced, all of her symptoms started to fade away. Today, Rachel is free from her "labels" and takes no medication.

The Future of Well Care

This book represents over a decade of working with complex, chronic illness. Through careful listening, hundreds of hours of research, and many humbling mistakes, I have been able to create a roadmap with clear guideposts that define patients as well or unwell and determine exactly how to recover them if they're not well. In other words, there is finally a three-dimensional under-standing for what's really happening within our bodies, a process we can optimize for our health when illness sets in.

Today, at The Gedroic Medical Institute, our ability to return chronically ill patients to their desired state of wellness is more than 90 percent when they are compliant with their treatment protocol, *regardless of their initial diagnoses, symptoms, and/or presentations or "labels."* We have worked with nearly every chronic condition in medicine today: all types of autoimmune disease, neurological conditions, chronic fatigue syndrome, fibromyalgia, attention deficit hyperactivity disorder (ADHD), behavioral disorders, depression, bipolar disorder, anxiety, and the list goes on. Once the body is defined with a new roadmap, it becomes clear that these diseases all represent dysregulated immune responses that are correctable.

We are meant to be well or we wouldn't have evolved for millions of years. **The basis of this book is that it *is* possible that the health of 90 percent of patients today can truly be recovered.** Instead of being "cured," I like to say that my patients have "lost their labels." I see this every day in my clinic. Patients who have spent ten, fifteen, or even twenty years with chronic illness routinely graduate to a state of wellness and are told to come back only if they ever need me again. Because of these successes, I believe wellness is truly within everyone's reach. But in order for this to happen, patients must demand knowledge of what is triggering their symptoms and underlying their diseases; each and every patient must challenge the current medical paradigm by asking "Why?" instead of accepting a prescription to treat only their symptoms.

The bottom line is that our medical and healthcare system is failing us today. We're at a crisis point now where we *must* change the trajectory of where healthcare is going and how healthcare professionals are treating disease for the sake of each and every patient who is not living their lives at 100 percent.

We do not have to accept disease diagnoses. We can maintain our health, free from symptoms, disease, drugs, and discomfort. It is not impossible to do so. We simply need to start looking at and approaching disease differently.

I hope you'll use this book as an inspiration to approach your own doctors about how to delve further into your health conditions, with the end goal of recovering your health for good. I hope you'll be the catalyst for change when it comes to your own health. Remember: Your health is in your own hands. Reclaiming control of your health and regaining the power over your own body is incredibly motivating. And if medicine can begin to look for the source of an illness, rather than merely treating its symptoms, we *can* stop the rising trend of chronic disease.

My patients have been my teachers, and my greatest hope is that this book will help all patients and doctors everywhere start to look at disease differently so we can change from A Nation of Unwell to A Nation of Well. I believe this can happen; it simply takes a sea change in how we view medicine. *A Nation of Unwell* is a guidebook for how and where to begin.

Kristine Gedroic, MD

PART I

A Nation of Unwell or Diagnosis Failure?

The part can never be well unless the whole is well.

—Plato

1

Chronic Sickness on the Rise, Despite Medical Advances

It's no medical secret that increasing numbers of people in America are becoming chronically sick. According to the Centers for Disease Control and Prevention (CDC), about half of all US adults (117 million people) have one or more chronic health conditions, and one in four US adults have two or more chronic health conditions. We also have a chronic sweep upward in the number of people taking prescription medications: nearly 60 percent of Americans, the highest number ever.[3]

At first glance, it might seem that because we are living longer and have more sophisticated diagnostics, people are being informed earlier about their health and are living longer with their conditions. This may be one small part of it, but it is not the complete picture. What is happening is that we as a nation are becoming sicker earlier, with new pediatric conditions being diagnosed more regularly than ever before. Almost 49 percent of Americans have taken at least one prescription medication in the past thirty days, while 23 percent of Americans have used three or more prescription drugs in order to just feel "well."[4] The average life expectancy is now for the first time lower in our generation than in previous generations. What is going on?

We as a nation are becoming weaker in our health and slowly but surely chronically unwell. How many people today know a child with a chronic diagnosis who will likely require medication in order to perform optimally in school or socially? Or a child who has a life-threatening allergy that prevents them from traveling safely without medication? Or an adult with a chronic inflammatory condition that requires long-term medication in order to maintain an optimal quality of life? This has sadly become the new normal—and it should not be. Because of this, as I've said, we must all take a step back from what's happening and ask in very simple terms, *Why?*

 FAST FACT Almost 22 percent of Americans have taken three or more prescription medications in the past thirty days in order to feel well, and the average life expectancy is now for the first time lower in our generation than in previous generations.

But first, let's take a look at some staggering statistics.

The CDC tells us that seven of the top ten causes of death are chronic diseases. Heart disease, ranked the number one cause of death in the United States, and cancer, ranked number two, are both on the rise. Both accounted for nearly 46 percent of all deaths. And what about the number of people diagnosed with and suffering from autoimmune diseases, conditions like type 1 diabetes, rheumatoid arthritis, psoriasis, lupus, celiac disease, and ulcerative colitis, which are all triggered by an abnormal immune response directed toward the body? Between twenty-four and fifty million Americans suffer from autoimmune diseases and these numbers have been rising steadily over the past thirty years.[5]

Then there are all the pediatric chronic conditions, such as ADHD, allergies, obesity, asthma, and learning and behavioral problems, that are on the rise. Now, nearly one out of four children (fifteen to eighteen million children aged seventeen or younger) live with chronic health conditions.[6] What on earth is going wrong? Children are simply not meant to have multiple medical conditions.

Think about this for a minute: despite an incredible wealth of healthcare resources—well-funded research, medical breakthroughs, powerful medications, and so much more—disease statistics are *still* on the rise in this country. What's more, patients keep getting diagnosed with new diseases, so-called "rare" or "orphan" diseases we've never heard of or never saw fifty or a hundred years ago.

Unfortunately, it's become the norm for us to live with and die from chronic disease. It saddens us but doesn't shock us anymore when we or a family member, friend, or colleague is diagnosed with breast cancer or any other type of cancer or chronic illness.

But I can't emphasize enough that this chronic state of unwell and disease is *not* normal. These statistics should make us all pause and question the status quo. This book will show how a successful model for change is within our reach.

The problem is not with our bodies, which may seem to be succumbing to debilitating disease at an alarming rate, but with the diagnosis and treatment of disease from the very start. The body is an incredibly dynamic organism, capable of fighting and overcoming most illnesses, as long as it has what it needs to do so. But our bodies are not getting what they need in terms of the proper nutrients, nourishment, and care. (See simple strategies to care for your body in "Your Two-Week Health-Boosting Plan," page 155.) In fact, we in America care for our cars better than we care for our own bodies.

The problem is with our current medical paradigm or model, which must start looking at symptoms as guides to what's happening in the body in order to point in the direction of true healing.

Most illnesses, with the exception of genetic diseases, are able to be reversed if addressed early, without a lifetime of drugs, simply by listening to the body's cries for help and by aiding the body in restoring its internal balance. Most of what is happening in medicine today is "epigenetic," meaning it develops from gestation over a lifetime.

This concept of epigenetics is an emerging but powerful concept in medicine today. Most patients believe that they suffer from "genetic conditions" like depression, high cholesterol, and/or high blood pressure. I hear every day in my practice: "Yes, my mother or father had high cholesterol; it runs in the family." But this does not mean it is inevitable or genetic.

Most of these conditions are "epigenetic," meaning that they occur independent of our DNA. When we're created, we receive a copy of DNA from our biological mother and a copy from our biological father. During gestation, this DNA and its ability to produce healthy genes are influenced by many factors, including Mom's nutrition, exposure to toxins, lifestyle, stress, and other factors. Once we are born, our DNA continues to be influenced by our environment in a similar way, and almost all modern disease states are the result of these processes affecting our genes, a concept known as epigenetics. Epigenetic conditions like high blood pressure, high cholesterol, type 2 diabetes, and depression can be treated and reversed since they have happened *to our DNA* and are not the direct result *of our DNA*. Most diseases are often the result of similar stressors or "epigenetic effects" occurring within families, with diet and lifestyle being key. It means that the same stressors on Mom or Dad are occurring in us, and our elevated blood pressure or elevated cholesterol, for example, is a reflection of that. It used to be that it took decades of stress on the human body before these conditions set in, but sadly, the onslaught of epigenetic effects is starting to affect us younger and younger with these conditions now on the rise in the pediatric population. We will delve further into the concept of epigenetics and modern stressors on the body later in this book.

HOW WE DIAGNOSE = DIAGNOSIS FAILURE

The downward spiral of health in America begins with the gold standard of diagnosis and treatment in America: Examine symptoms and blood work to label a condition, ignoring the potential for reversal; then, prescribe medication, sometimes a drug designed to be taken for the rest of one's life, to treat the symptoms. This is the paradigm of health and illness today.

This is not normal and should not be accepted as normal.

Let's consider, for example, that Mrs. Jones shows up at the doctor with a history of acid reflux: burning pain in her lower chest, dry coughing that doesn't go away, and regular reflux after meals. Her doctor tells her, "You have GERD (gastroesophageal reflux disease). Take this pill daily to help you get back to your life without discomfort."

Mrs. Jones is relieved; she finally has a label for the symptoms she's been experiencing (*I have GERD*) and begins medication, which prevents the symptoms from occurring. Like Mrs. Jones, so many of us are our labels:

I am healthy if I feel well and have no medical label.

I am sick if I feel unwell and have a label (e.g., I have IBS).

I am okay if I have a label and a medicine helps me feel better. (I take medication, which is helping control my IBS. I am feeling healthy again.)

A glaring omission is a questioning of why the symptoms are occurring in the first place. Why does Mrs. Jones have acid reflux at all? When and why did it start? And why, despite being on medication, has it gotten progressively worse, sometimes affecting her ability to work, care for her family, and live a vibrant life?

This labeling of conditions and diseases, without an in-depth probing of why they're occurring, is actually *mislabeling,* and it's one of the key reasons why we are where we are today with our healthcare and with chronic illness and disease spiraling out of control.

The current linear medical paradigm, Symptom A = Syndrome B = Medicine C, is *incorrect.* Medicine C may help diminish or take away Symptom A, but it doesn't resolve or "cure" Syndrome B. Instead of saying, "I get acid reflux after I eat" (a description of symptoms), Mrs. Jones can now tell herself and anyone who asks, "I have GERD and I'm taking drug X to fix it." Drug X will help ease Mrs. Jones's symptoms and make her feel better, but it won't address the root cause of her illness; it also won't address what her body needs in order to heal itself.

For example, why might a patient be experiencing chronic sleeplessness? It's easy to prescribe a drug to force the body to fall asleep; it's much harder to figure out why the sleeplessness is occurring in the first place. The same is true for indigestion, chronic pain, fatigue, skin rashes, persistent acne, chronic congestion, migraines, GERD, and the list goes on. These symptoms are just the tip of the so-called health iceberg; it's what these symptoms mean that is the crux of why the body is out of balance.

But when no diagnosis is made, then what? Unlike Mrs. Jones with her GERD diagnosis, there are plenty of people who leave a doctor's office *without* a diagnosis in hand. Their clinical symptoms and blood work don't point to any one condition or label, so the patient might hear, "Well, Mr. Smith, it sounds like you have diagnosis X, but your tests don't show this. In fact, you seem to have no condition or illness. Your tests are coming up quite normal."

But Mr. Smith doesn't feel normal. He goes home with a drug or drugs prescribed by the doctor to quell his symptoms, but he never really feels well. How many people have heard a loved one or friend told, despite daily suffering, that nothing is wrong with them. There are no statistics on the number of people who walk around with symptoms, sometimes debilitating, that are undiagnosed. Yet most of us know someone in our immediate household or close family and friends who suffer from some chronic symptom that has no real cause, so they simply live with it. If it gets bad enough, they will ultimately seek out a doctor and qualify for medication, possibly a pain medication, which hopefully makes living with the symptom more manageable but never truly resolves it.

Or even worse: "Mr. Smith, since your labs are all normal and you still feel unwell, I think you're depressed and should see a psychiatrist." My question in response: What is this conclusion being based on? The fact that the labs are all "normal" and therefore there is nothing medically wrong, so it must be in the patient's head? Many of these "depressed" patients have what I refer to as a biological cause of their depression (e.g., an infection or toxin) and can be recovered without a lifetime of mood-stabilizing drugs.

The reality is that the entire medical model as it exists today must change if we want to change the trajectory of chronic disease. The tests that are being used to analyze or "work up" patients are not giving doctors the needed information to help patients recover. Once we start to define health differently—and we can, as you'll see—we will be able to clearly identify what is at the root of chronic disease and begin to help patients recover their wellness long term.

SYMPTOMS: HOW OUR BODY COMMUNICATES

When patients don't feel well, their symptoms—most of the time—tell the whole story. A patient with gastrointestinal (GI) distress, for instance, has an imbalance in their intestines. Their distress is manifested in symptoms like bloating, pain, and a change in bowel patterns before and after meals. These are all the symptoms that help guide us to the underlying disturbance.

When I meet with patients, they tell me their unique story (including their symptoms), how the symptoms started, and the journey they've had, along with how they feel today, which is invariably not great. This all holds the clues to why they are no longer well.

Healing from chronic disease is like peeling back the layers of an onion. This is why I ask patients to tell me everything, since nothing in the body is unrelated. It is often the unrelated elements of the story that hold the real truth.

As physicians, though, we are not trained to consider *why* patients are having symptoms in an attempt to correct the underlying cause. We are taught to ask the questions we need to have answered in order to add up to a particular disease or diagnosis, and we are trained to consider what medicine will help with the symptom and make the patient more comfortable or less at risk. We then discard all the other elements that seem to have no relation. But true learning about health happens in the inverse. What makes sense is the easy part; it's the parts that don't add up that point us to what's really going on in the body. Despite years of learning, I still don't always know why a patient feels a certain way, but his/her symptoms steer me in the direction of the research I need to do to better explain the cause of the symptoms and in time, guide the body back to wellness.

What we are taught in medical school also fails to emphasize the powerful underlying principle of health, the fact that the systems within our bodies have evolved to work in harmony and are set up to self-regulate. In other words, we are all capable of truly healing, which most of the time starts in the gut. The basic essence of health is that the body is always attempting to arc toward balance and wellness. The body wants to be healthy and is capable of being healthy without a lifetime of medications.

The bottom line is, patients need to be looked at for the unique individuals they are and managed in a comprehensive way. We are so much more as a whole than the sum of our parts. Much, much more.

What Symptoms Are Telling Us

Symptoms are the way the body communicates to us the kind of stress it's under. Another way to look at what's going on in our bodies is to imagine that we are all born with a figurative "sink" that is able to accommodate stressors—from our food, water, personal care products, and environment. This sink is bigger or smaller depending on our genes, and how we lead our lives affects how quickly the sink fills up (the concept of epigenetics). Those of us who live cleanly have sinks that fill up slowly, if ever. Those of us who don't take care of ourselves are quick to fill our sinks, which will inevitably overflow. There is also the small percentage of us who genetically have "large sinks" and despite not living clean or eating well seem to escape most illnesses.

FAST FACT Another way to look at what's going on in our bodies is to imagine that we are all born with a figurative "sink" that is able to accommodate stressors—from our food, water, personal care products, and environment. This sink is bigger or smaller depending on our genes, and how we lead our lives affects how quickly the sink fills up (the concept of epigenetics).

When this sink starts to overflow, we develop symptoms like headaches/migraines, pain, digestive upset (bloating, gas, belching, acid reflux, constipation, diarrhea), insomnia, depression, anxiety/irritability, chronic congestion, achy joints, mood swings, persistent acne, eczema (and other skin conditions), hormonal imbalance, allergies/asthma, and lack of energy/fatigue, to name just a few.

Symptoms are our bodies' cries for help, which, if not interpreted correctly, can go on for years, even decades, before chronic disease sets in. They are the body's way of signaling to us that something isn't right, that something is out of balance. The body is always striving to achieve wellness or balance. When it needs help from the outside, it sends out a signal in the form of symptoms.

In fact, symptoms are the *only* way for our incredible and powerful bodies to communicate with us. Instead of stopping to listen to these symptoms and try to understand what's causing them, we instead readily take a pill to silence the symptoms. Once silenced, it is only a matter of time before the body cries out with yet another symptom, and another, in an attempt to call attention to, with increased urgency, its state of imbalance, which is readily getting worse.

I liken this scenario to the fire and smoke detector analogy I shared earlier. When we take medicine for a symptom without looking for a cause, we are dismantling our internal smoke detector while the fire continues to burn, becoming more intense and problematic over time. Once all these symptoms have been ignored or silenced for good with medications, the body finally succumbs, worn out, to disease. Once disease sets in, our natural sink has already effectively overflowed.

Of course, medication is necessary at times to ease acute symptoms, and under these circumstances I will prescribe what's necessary for a patient. But all of the time, I am trying to determine the root cause of a patient's symptom/s and how I can get them back into balance long term without medication.

This is why I love symptoms: they are the clues I need to begin a patient's roadmap to wellness. The more symptoms, the clearer I am about what the body is trying to say.

The first step is to understand what the body's system or particular organ is trying to tell us; the next step is to figure out the most efficient way to fix it and heal the patient. A headache hurts and is inconvenient, for example, but it is the way the body tells us to drink more (and cleaner) water; stop eating gluten or dairy or another food you're sensitive to; or even something more serious, such as there's too much mold in your home and you need to find a way to remediate it, fast.

We need to start considering these symptoms as the body's cries for help. Symptoms are not merely something to medicate and extinguish. **Symptoms are to be honored for what they are telling us. Think of the power and beauty in that: Our bodies can't talk to us in words. They talk to us in symptoms.** We simply need to start listening to get a glimpse of what's going on inside the body and, more specifically, inside our cells.

WHAT A HEALTHY CELL LOOKS LIKE

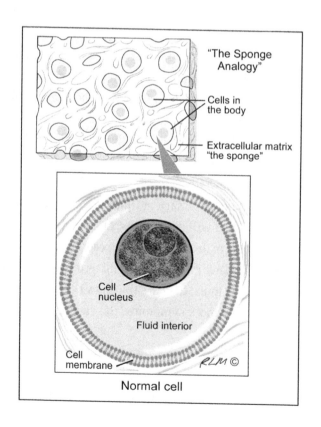

Our bodies are made up of cells, trillions and trillions of cells of different shapes and sizes. (One estimate put the number of cells in the body at 37.2 trillion.[7]) Thousands of new cells are replicated daily, replacing the old damaged cells. These are what all your tissues and organs are made from. If these cells are healthy, we are healthy. If these cells are unhealthy, we experience illness and disease.

What exactly is a healthy cell and what makes it healthy?

Take a deep breath in and a long, slow breath out. As we breathe in, we take in critical oxygen. As we breathe out, we exhale waste in the form of carbon dioxide. Cells are no different. All cells are surrounded by an outside protective porous cell membrane comprised mainly of fats and some proteins. Healthy cells are able to take in nutrients through this porous membrane, which is between four and ten nanometers thick, and eliminate waste through this membrane. (To put this cellular membrane in perspective, it would take about 10,000 membranes to make up the thickness of one sheet of paper.[8]) Cells are in continuous interaction with each other through something called the extracellular matrix, communicating and working together for the health of an organ or the body as a whole.

The extracellular matrix is an area in the body that I liken to a sponge, which is why I refer to this concept as "The Sponge Analogy." I ask patients to imagine our cells as the holes of a sponge. The extracellular matrix is the actual sponge, apart from the holes, that connects all the cells in the body. It's extremely important to keep our "sponges" clean since the matrix is what allows for optimal cell-to-cell communication and protects us from having toxins (stressors) enter our cells and potentially affect our DNA. The matrix is where chemical toxins—from our food, water, personal care products, home cleaning products, and environment—get stored until the liver or kidneys have a chance to detoxify them. If the matrix is congested and "toxic," however, these toxins begin to pass through the cell wall, making their way into the inner part of our cells where they attach to the DNA, creating an epigenetic event. This is the beginning of many of the health issues we are seeing in medicine today.

I find this sponge analogy helps patients visualize what's happening inside their cells so they can better understand where a healthy, or an unhealthy, body starts from. It also helps to emphasize why the concept of "toxicity" is so important in recovering a patient from chronic illness to a state of well.

Symptoms occur when the body and cellular health is out of balance and desperately needs to get back into balance. If cells don't have enough balancers (e.g., the right minerals, vitamins, fats, and proteins) to outweigh the stressors that the body is dealing with (see more in Chapter 5 on page 127), they become depleted and unable to stay healthy. If they do have enough balancers, all systems within the body are working in harmony, and the body is able to fight off everyday illness and resist disease. Disease occurs when stressors or acquired toxins outweigh the body's balancers. As such, diseases don't develop in only one day.

Consider this: there are people we all know who get a cold, produce mucus, cough a lot, blow their nose, and then get over it. This is the body's natural response to a toxin or virus when its cellular health is in balance. In an individual whose cellular health is depleted, however, and whose symptoms along the way have been ignored, he may within a few days get pneumonia from a simple virus and require medication to even survive. This is a person with what is called a depleted constitution, which means his body is not able to overcome a normal toxic burden. In order to heal him, we would need to understand and treat his underlying symptoms, then strengthen his constitution in order for him to once again be healthy. After that, he would easily recover from a common cold, other virus, or even bacterial infection that comes his way.

Through my experience with thousands of people in my medical practice, I have found that fixing the underlying imbalance in the body and the cells prevents and, yes, even *reverses* chronic disease. In fixing the overflowing sink, with all its problems, we allow people to live healthy and disease-free (and prescription medicine–free) for years to come.

We *must* rethink our approach to health if we are to stem the rising tide of chronic disease in America, and we *must* return the body to a state of being well by balancing out this health seesaw. It *is* possible. In my clinic, I have successfully done this time and time again with chronically ill patients. These same patients end up becoming symptom-free and disease-free.

Does this mean that I'm the only doctor who can ever treat these chronically ill patients, the only doctor who can make sick people well? No. Every single doctor and patient can do this by delving deep to understand why the symptoms are occurring in the first place. This is how together, as a medical team, we can unravel the mystery of what the body is communicating to us. And this is how we can put an end to the disturbing upward trajectory of chronic disease.

Doctors are not and should not be the miracle workers. Each and every one of our bodies is the miracle worker, telling us what's wrong with them. We simply have to learn to listen to what our bodies are telling us. And that's exactly what I'll show you how to do throughout this book.

RYAN'S STORY

A concerned mother came in to see me with her ten-year-old son, Ryan. He had persistent, severe eczema on both arms and legs that itched so much he had scabs from the scratching. Needless to say, he was also unable to sleep because of all the itching. He had already been to see multiple doctors who were not able to diagnose why he was so sick and why he was not getting better. The last doctor Ryan had seen had recommended that he start a chemotherapy drug, methotrexate, to calm down what he considered to be his overactive immune system.

Ryan's mom felt in her gut that this was wrong. That's when she brought Ryan to see me. The real questions that should have been asked about Ryan were: *Why would his system be behaving like this? What is really going on?*

In sitting down to talk with Ryan's mother and examine him, I asked my usual questions that delve into a patient's background, environment, diet, mother's pregnancy, and more. In my years working with patients, I have found that every question and every patient's answer is relevant to the state of their health now. Since Ryan's eczema was not responding to the traditional immunosuppressive therapies for allergic reactions, I suspected that an epigenetic event was underlying his eczema. In other words, a toxin was causing his body to be in a chronic state of inflammation. An epigenetic cause would be largely unresponsive to traditional therapies for eczema, as was the case with Ryan.

As it turns out, Ryan's school was downwind from a superfund site that had been recently compromised during a hurricane. (Superfund sites are areas contaminated by hazardous waste and are designated as such by the Environmental Protection Agency.) Ever since that time, Ryan's school had been repeatedly closed for high levels of toxic air. That is when Ryan's eczema began.

What testing ultimately revealed was that Ryan did in fact have a toxin causing his eczema, which we were able to resolve with a liver support and detoxification treatment protocol. In hindsight, it's a good thing Ryan's mom thought twice about allowing Ryan to take a chemotherapy drug, since suppressing Ryan's immune system was not at all what his body needed. What Ryan's body *did* need was for us to stop, listen to what it was telling us, and give it the necessary tools to get healthy on its own. Today, Ryan remains free from eczema. He is a healthy young boy who I now see only once a year for wellness checks.

MICHAEL'S STORY

Michael is a young adult who spent four years in a state of chronic and almost debilitating fatigue before he came to see me. He was constantly exhausted, having little energy to do his college work, hang out with friends, or do much of anything.

I found out, over the course of my questioning, that Michael had a wet basement that had never been checked for mold. All indoor molds, not merely the proverbial "black mold," are toxic to the body. When in an indoor environment, molds often produce mycotoxins (toxic chemicals produced by fungi) that disrupt the barrier function of the gastrointestinal or GI tract, causing liver inflammation, neurological disease, liver damage, and much more. What's more, these mycotoxins are easily spread around homes with forced-air heating systems.

Prior to the mid-twentieth century, most people relied on radiator heat to keep their homes warm. For this reason, if molds were growing in their basements, they didn't pose as much of a health threat because they weren't easily spread. The use of lead paint also stopped the growth of mold, as lead is an antifungal. Once lead paint was phased out and forced-air heating systems were on the rise, more and more people began to get sick from indoor mold.

In Michael's case, his forced-air heating system was circulating the mold throughout his home. As he breathed it in, he became sicker. The sicker he got, the more time he spent at home, and the more he became affected by the mold toxins. It was, and is for many, a vicious cycle.

Anyone exposed to mold toxins or mycotoxins on a regular basis can become critically ill, particularly those whose cellular "sink" is on the verge of overflowing. Mycotoxins fill our proverbial sink very quickly because of the damage they cause to the body. They are powerful neurotoxins and are the trigger behind many neurological symptoms like headaches, blurry vision, numbness and tingling, mild tremors, persistent anxiety, and sensitivity to noise and light. These same toxins can also cause gastrointestinal complaints like nausea and vomiting, rashes, and chronic fatigue. This is a growing area of research, but more studies still need to be done to determine exactly how and why these mycotoxins affect people differently.

FAST FACT Mycotoxins fill our proverbial sink very quickly because of the damage they cause to the body. They are powerful neurotoxins and are the trigger behind many neurological symptoms like headaches, blurry vision, numbness and tingling, mild tremors, persistent anxiety, and sensitivity to noise and light. These same toxins can also cause gastrointestinal complaints like nausea and vomiting, rashes, and chronic fatigue.

Anyone who tells you that mold in your home (if present) isn't affecting your health isn't looking at the whole picture. The body simply cannot do its job staying healthy when it's being inundated with mycotoxins. Michael's mold levels and mycotoxins were some of the highest I had ever seen.

In Michael's case, no one had correlated the significant demise of his health with where he was spending time: in a home with a moldy basement. Once we uncovered this critical health clue, as we have for hundreds of patients, Michael had a much clearer path to recovery. He had his basement tested and discovered that the mold levels were, predictably, extremely high. After his basement was cleared of the mold through a licensed mold remediation company, I put him on a treatment protocol for mold exposure and detoxification, and I gave him the nutritional supplements he needed to repair his cellular functioning.

Today, Michael is back at college and holding a part-time job. Now, with no medication, he is one of our graduates living a normal life. He continues to take some basic nutrients and, as we all should do, eats a clean diet to keep his body healthy, nothing more.

MY OWN STORY

I'm passionate about helping my patients recover since I've lived through my own health crisis. I know the labels that were given to me and the challenges I faced on my road to full recovery. It is not a coincidence that I now feel it is my purpose to help my patients regain their health with the clear direction I did not have.

At age twenty-eight, having just graduated from medical school with a spot in a coveted plastic surgery residency at Weill Cornell Medical Center in

New York City, my health started deteriorating after only the first year. I was working more than a hundred hours a week, and I chalked up the frequent, debilitating migraines I was getting to simply being stressed and having a lot on my plate. I also chalked up my newly diagnosed gastric ulcer to the same cause. After all, I had just run a marathon, so I was in "excellent" health.

What I didn't realize is that my own sink was starting to overflow.

I thought nothing of taking prescription migraine pills and acid blockers, which, in hindsight, were merely stifling my body's cries for help. What began as medication to treat the occasional migraine, though, soon became daily pills that stopped getting results. I began to rotate from one medication to the next. Nothing seemed to work because I wasn't addressing the underlying causes, only I didn't realize this at the time.

It's important to mention here that during this period, none of the doctors I consulted asked me about my diet. I was living on diet soda made with the chemical sweetener aspartame to stay awake, along with whole wheat bagels that I stashed in my white doctor's coat and nibbled on all day long for energy. Years later, when I finally discovered my triggers for migraines (which ironically turned out to be gluten, dairy, and aspartame), I realized that removing these foods from my diet would have made my life, and my health, infinitely better back then. These same foods were also affecting my stomach and were part of what needed to change in order for my stomach to heal. But incredibly, not one single doctor ever asked what I was eating. By continuing to eat and live the way I was, along with taking prescription medicines, I was ignoring what my body really needed.

Soon my body's cries for help got louder and, not surprisingly, my medical condition got worse, eventually spiraling out of control.

One of the medications I was taking had a severe, almost fatal, side effect. Along with a series of ensuing serious complications, I found myself, the marathon-running surgical resident in "perfect health," in the ICU.

That's when I realized how wrong my reality was. I decided to step away from medicine. *After all*, I thought, *the medicines I had grown to know and love had almost taken my life, so what was I to believe in anymore?* I retreated to my parents' home in New Jersey where I grew up, and it wasn't until my mother took me to see a nearby integrative physician that my health started to turn around.

This integrative doctor examined my diet, my daily routines, and my life and determined that changing these things, as well as taking some critical supplements, would transform my health. And it did, dramatically. Within only a few days, I was feeling stronger and healthier and had more energy. My migraines and stomach problems slowly stopped. Today I can eat gluten and even certain forms of dairy, but only for a few days at a time. When the old symptoms start to return, I am reminded of how beautiful our bodies are at letting us know when enough is enough.

Once full recovery was in sight, I decided to put my sights on a business degree in medical biotechnology. Two days before the GMAT, however, and now many months after leaving my surgical residency at Cornell, I went to dinner with my family. In the midst of our meal, a woman at the table next to us slumped over and became unconscious. No one knew what had happened, but I jumped into action and began CPR. The twelve months of acute, critical care in New York hospitals had created an instinct in me of which I was unaware. I realized then that medicine was my true calling and I needed to go back, only on different terms. The woman, who had lapsed into a diabetic coma, did survive. I'm grateful I had the instincts and the knowledge to help her at that moment. And I'm grateful to her for unknowingly helping me steer my career back to medicine.

It was after this incident that I enrolled in a family practice residency at Overlook Hospital in Summit, New Jersey, the hospital where I was born. I knew then that I needed to share my knowledge about blending the best of medicine with the integrative strategies that had ultimately healed me. But I didn't have the slightest clue how to begin. There was no example for me to follow of the practice I wanted to create. I simply knew that if I continued to follow my passion and practice the best medicine I knew how, the answer would come. And it did.

As I neared the end of my residency, I was inspired to train in acupuncture, so I pursued a medical acupuncture degree at New York Medical College and two years later took the Medical Acupuncture Boards. I also became inspired by integrative medicine pioneer Dr. Andrew Weil. I was regularly using his DVDs and CDs to learn the proper breath work during meditation, something that I had started doing to stay balanced and de-stressed. I ultimately pursued a fellowship at The University of Arizona Center for Integrative Medicine, founded by Dr. Weil and where he still serves as director.

This was the most important step I made on my journey to a new form of medicine. I finally had a framework by which to organize all of the natural healing methods I had come to know and embrace from my own healing and through my own research. More importantly, I realized there was a whole community of like-minded doctors. I had an instant network of support and camaraderie, which was motivating and was the jump-start I needed to open a small family practice, one that grew and became focused on integrative health.

Today, my clinic is called The Gedroic Medical Institute, and we see and recover some of the most complex medical issues people face. The work can be extremely challenging, but each case teaches me even more about the beauty of the human body and how gracefully it can recover if given the proper tools. The cases we see are truly transformative. Children with severe allergies, behavioral disorders, and chronic gastrointestinal complaints become well without medication. Young women and men with autoimmune diseases, chronic fatigue, and neurological disorders have their conditions reversed. They never have to take medication again, and they go on to have healthy lives. Adults with chronic pain, fatigue, and depression recover and are once again able to enjoy life to the fullest. Over the years, these patients have been the consummate teachers. I have had to study each case and develop individualized roadmaps to recovery, but each recovery started with listening to what they and their bodies were telling me. Everything I've learned with each and every patient, I've used with subsequent patients. It has truly been a yellow brick road of learning with a goal of wellness for all as the driving force. To be able to assist my patients on their journey to wellness is a gift I never could have imagined.

EMPOWERED TO STAY HEALTHY

Once our health graduates heal, they never become what I call chronic patients. They're energized again about living and being healthy. They learn to respect their bodies, guided by listening to what their bodies are telling them and eating and drinking well in order to stay healthy. Why? Because this is part of the healing and recovery process that we send home with each patient. Health is back in the patient's hands, where it should be. This message is incredibly powerful and motivating.

Each and every one of us is strong and capable of being healthy. But many patients cycle from doctor to doctor, getting prescription drug after prescription drug to treat their symptoms, without anyone ever getting to the heart of the health problem and why the symptoms are occurring in the first place.

FAST FACT

Each and every one of us is strong and capable of being healthy. But many patients cycle from doctor to doctor, getting prescription drug after prescription drug to treat their symptoms, without anyone ever getting to the heart of the health problem and why the symptoms are occurring in the first place.

This dependency on drugs creates a vulnerability in the mind of chronically ill patients: *There's something wrong with me. My body has failed me. I'll never be healthy.* No wonder depression is a common side effect of chronic illness. Nothing, though, could be further from the truth. The bodies of these patients are doing exactly what they need to do by communicating through symptoms like depression, which most of the time is another signal of a body out of balance.

A patient's loss of faith in their own body is a negativity, I believe, that contributes to the state of chronic disease. There's also an attitude of, *Oh well, I might as well eat whatever I want because I figured out what was wrong with me and now have a drug, or medical procedure, to fix it.*

Confidence in what the body can do is something I try to give back to each of my patients: I empower them to care for and listen to their bodies so that once they get better, they can stay healthy. This can be done by eating a clean diet with little to no processed foods, artificial sweeteners, or sugar (which depresses the immune system, making it unable to stay healthy); exercising regularly; getting enough sleep; and encouraging positive emotions and a healthy spirit. (For simple, doable daily tips on how to be healthy, see "Your Two-Week Health-Boosting Plan," page 155.)

In the next chapter, I'm going to talk about how medicine got to where we are today, why the current approach may have worked at its inception in the early 1900s, and how it needs to and can change for the better moving forward.

2

The Evolution of Medicine: How We Got Where We Are Today

How did we get so sick? How did we become a nation of the chronically unwell despite all the tremendous advances we've made in medicine? Think about it. We are a nation of the most sophisticated medical advances and cutting-edge diagnostics and treatments. And yet the average person today is still unwell in some way. Why is this? The answer lies in the evolution of society and why medicine must now change in order to keep up. The way in which healers, doctors, and trained professionals have interpreted and treated illness and disease for thousands of years is falling short today; we need a new model.

Medicine's sole purpose, from the beginning of civilization, has been to get people well and to transform sickness into health. But now something is profoundly wrong. Despite all the years of medical research we have under our proverbial belt and the access patients now have to tremendous healthcare advances, people aren't getting well. They're getting sicker and they're staying that way.

Despite all the years of medical research we have under our proverbial belt and the access patients now have to tremendous healthcare advances, people aren't getting well. They're getting sicker and they're staying that way.

GENETICALLY WIRED TO BE HEALTHY

Since the earliest days of humanity, people were either born healthy or born with a genetic illness or condition. You were well or you weren't; it was as simple as that. And if you weren't well, you could be healed with a variety of plant-based medicines or rudimentary "treatments," or you died a quick death. There were no lingering illnesses that lasted years; this was true even though people lived shorter lives. The fact that people are living longer now means our bodies have much longer periods of time in which to contract disease. A shorter lifespan can't completely account for the lack of chronic illness and disease in the past. Something more was at play then.

Disease in our early history typically occurred only when we faced famine, were maimed, or suffered a life-threatening bacterial or viral infection (of which there have been many throughout the years). Some diseases were brought on by animals and bugs like mosquitos; others were brought on by poor nutrition, lack of necessary nutrients like vitamin C, and unsanitary conditions.

Treatment was straightforward: patients had an imbalance in the body that needed to be corrected. In early medicine, which dominated treatment until the late 1800s, healing an imbalance of the humors (or principal fluids in the body) was the key to solving any illness in the body. These fluids—black bile, yellow bile, phlegm, and blood—were produced by the body's organs and needed to be in harmony, doctors believed, for the body to be well. Diet (including plants and herbs), early medicines, and bloodletting were typically used to create parity among these principal fluids in the body and return the body to health. (During bloodletting, a medical "doctor," or sometimes even a barber surgeon[9], nicked a vein with a crude lancet or sharpened piece of wood to let the blood flow out.) Thankfully, we've come a long way from this primitive medical treatment, but in doing so, we've also gotten away from the simple idea of equilibrium in the body. In other words, a balanced body is a healthy one, a concept that I mention many times throughout this book.

As travel and colonization increased, more sicknesses like malaria, diphtheria, smallpox, and yellow fever were spread among people living closer together. Small-town physicians, as well as preachers, midwives, and "healers," all of whom were the trusted medical professionals of their day, administered care. At this time, the medical theory of healing the body by balancing out the humors still dominated. Patients were "cured" by purging, vomiting, blistering, and/or bleeding or bloodletting, all meant to correct an imbalance in the body or let the "demons" out, as some doctors believed.[10]

As crude as bloodletting was, and is, it was the mainstream "healing" method until the advent of modern medicine. In theory, bloodletting and balancing the humors in the body were based on the fundamental idea that a sick patient's body had too much of something in it and needed to be rebalanced in order to be healthy again. While bloodletting is not something that needs to be reintroduced to our medical system, the important theory behind it has been lost in today's medical paradigm. This theory, that illness often represents too much of something that shouldn't be there, does need to be reintroduced. It is one I use every day with my own patients, and it is an important part of each patient's return to wellness.

PLANT-BASED MEDICINE = EARLY PHARMACEUTICALS

Another method of healing that dates back thousands of years is using plants and their bark, seeds, berries, and/or leaves to heal the body, curing illness and alleviating pain. There's evidence dating back five thousand years that Sumerians used more than 250 plants, including poppy and mandrake, to heal the body. These plants were the earliest "drugs." Over the years, every single culture has reached out to the plants around them for answers. In fact, while the American colonists were using bloodletting, the Native Americans were living off the plants that grew around them to stay healthy. These included plants like *lomatium dissectum* (also known as desert parsley), echinacea, and goldenseal. In fact, during the flu pandemic of 1918, only one group was reported to fare better than everyone else: the Native Americans in Nevada who used *lomatium dissectum* as a powerful herbal antiviral.[11] For those who relied on herbs and plants, which were the only remedies they had, the plants that got results were passed down through the generations as medical treatments.

As we entered the world of modern medicine, many of these "proven" plants became the basis for modern drugs: aspirin comes from the bark of a willow tree, which contains salicylic acid (Hippocrates recommended chewing on the bark of a willow tree to reduce fever as far back as 300 BC); morphine and codeine are based on active ingredients found in the opium poppy; Sudafed was developed from a bush called the ephedra sinica (also called ma-huang in Traditional Chinese Medicine); and penicillin was created from a mold called penicillin mold. Even the modern anticancer drug Taxol was developed from the Pacific yew tree, or *Taxus brevifolia.*[12]

While herbal concoctions were prepared for years from the plants themselves, modern-day chemists began to extract the active molecules from plants to make modern-day drugs in a lab. With the advent of these medical drugs, doctors and patients began to rely solely on these drugs for healing, with the actual plants and their usefulness relegated to questionable "alternative" therapies. In so doing, this rise of modern medicine created a new paradigm that was simple and linear. One was well until they became ill; and when they became ill, medical drugs created in a lab (not treatments from nature) could fix them.

Slowly, medicine and more specifically pharmaceutical drugs became the new answer to staying well. Again, without a genetic defect, most people were well until they became sick. When they became sick, they went to the doctor, who now had the ability to prescribe a medication that would "fix" the problem and was, by definition, more powerful than any home remedy. In both the doctors' and patients' minds, drugs became necessary for health.

Anything other than pharmaceuticals began to be referred to as "alternative," despite the fact that various other models of medicine with herbalism at their core have been practiced far longer than the drug-based medicine that is practiced today.

The problem today is that illness is no longer a linear relationship with only "one thing" causing "one disease." Most ongoing health conditions today are due to chronic inflammation, which is a conglomerate of various stressors on the body. In other words, it is more than "one thing," and there is no "one medicine" that is going to change it. We have to start unraveling illness at its core and, ideally, at its inception (i.e., gestation, infancy, and childhood) in order to help the next generation do better with healthcare than we're doing today.

Sickness today is the result of a body becoming seriously out of balance, as I'll detail more in coming chapters. The medicines of today do amazing things for acute symptoms and save millions of lives in the short term, but national averages tell us we need to start doing better in the long term. Medicine today is correcting the symptoms, not the source of illness. Constipated? *A new drug will help that problem.* Got insomnia? *Take this pill, and you'll be able to sleep through the night.* Have an itchy, persistent skin rash? *Use this prescription cream and it will go away.* Have unrelenting acne? *Take this prescription to make it disappear.*

 The medicines of today do amazing things for acute symptoms and save millions of lives in the short term, but national averages tell us we need to start doing better in the long term. Medicine today is correcting the symptoms, not the source of illness.

Once the symptoms go away with the help of drugs, other symptoms eventually crop up in their place as the body continues to cry out for help. Add to these symptoms the drugs' side effects, which are often treated with other prescription drugs. Now you can understand why people's figurative sinks are literally overflowing. Over time, this leads to even greater problems and chronic imbalance or "dis-ease."

The bigger issue is our psychological comfort with taking medication to maintain wellness without asking the question *Why?* This is illustrated most in our children. Why should children need a pill to be happy or to focus on homework, without first exploring the effect of their lifestyle, diet, and the environment around them? Today, it is quite normal for children to be taking daily medications for symptoms that begin in the early years of life. It is our society's mindset of dependence on medical drugs for wellness that we *must* break to slow down the rapid rise of chronic illness and disease in this country.

THE MODERN CAUSES OF ILLNESS

Hundreds of years ago, people lived simply off the sea and/or land, where they grew their own food and raised their own chickens and livestock. There was no modern refrigeration or bacterial control. In fact, before the advent of refrigeration, all cultures had ways of adding bacteria to foods in order to preserve them naturally at room temperatures, where these foods could safely stay "fresh" for weeks to months. These were the earliest probiotics. And this is where most condiments consumed today, such as mustard, chutney, pickles, kimchi, and sauerkraut, had their beginnings. These condiments were consumed with meals and unintentionally aided digestion by repopulating the gastrointestinal tract with healthy bacteria.

When there was no industrialization, there were also no processed convenience foods. There were no chemicals like pesticides and herbicides, also called biocides, added to our food supply. Food was clean, with no chemicals in it or on it. For this reason, diseases were singular and limited to specific, singular causes (bacteria in food and surroundings, unsanitary conditions, vector-borne illnesses like malaria and yellow fever, and lack of nutrition). I say this not to idealize the arduous conditions of our ancestors but to emphasize that life was very different then. And ironically people were, as a result, less prone to the kind of modern chronic, lingering diseases and illnesses we're witness to today.

Once industrialization began, a whole host of new health issues arose for these reasons:

• **Overcrowding** Once colonies were formed, the rise of infectious diseases increased. The closer people live together, the more likely they are to catch whatever disease someone else has. Once towns and cities were settled—before, during, and after the Industrial Revolution—infectious diseases like typhoid spread rapidly, infecting and often killing thousands of people. In the late 1800s and early 1900s, infectious respiratory diseases like pneumonia and TB were top threats to health. Infectious gastrointestinal diseases like cholera and typhoid also afflicted scores of people through contaminated food and water.

As people flocked to cities, they were likely to suffer from health problems as a result of living in close proximity to others and from breathing in the unfiltered pollution from factories. There's simply no substitute for fresh air when it comes to health, which brings me to my next point.

• **Toxins in the Environment** As we continued to evolve, so too did the rise of factories and industrialization. People began to suffer from ills that resulted from the accumulation of toxins in both their work and home environments. Coalminer's lung developed in those exposed to coal fumes. Factory pollution created smog (a combination of smoke and fog) and that—along with tar, soot, and ash spewed into the air—triggered lung irritation, chronic bronchitis, and pneumonia. (Tar in the air can incapacitate the lungs.[13]) Drinking water and farm runoff water were often polluted as factories—without any kind of regulation—dumped pollutants directly into rivers and streams. Water contained contaminants like heavy metals, sewage, and the toxic waste from factories, often referred to as toxic sludge.

The rise of the automobile escalated breathing difficulties and pollution in the air. A recent review of research found that breathing in too much car and truck exhaust can increase the risk of asthma, serious respiratory diseases later in life, and even cardiac problems.[14] This modern research can be extrapolated to the early twentieth century and the rise of the automobile, which contained even more toxins than the current exhaust today, a result of much-needed pollution regulations.

Case in point: it was in 1923 that something called tetraethyl lead was added to gasoline to improve a car's performance. Now, in addition to the pollution from exhaust, lead—a neurotoxin that accumulates in the brain, liver, kidneys, and bones—was continually being expelled into the air. And, because lead doesn't break down in the air, it began to be deposited in the soil and on the ground, tracked into homes, and ingested. (Lead was also added to paint in the early 1900s, so bodies were getting bombarded with lead's toxic effects both indoors and out.) Lead has been proven to interfere with nervous system development and contributes to behavioral disorders, convulsions, kidney damage, hypertension, and reproductive organ toxicity.[15] In pregnant women, lead exposure has been shown to cause miscarriage, stillbirths, premature births, and low-birthweight babies.

Lead toxicity was a problem then and is still a problem in areas around the country like Flint, Michigan, where lead leached into the water supply through old, corroded lead pipes. (Yes, drinking water actually flowed through lead pipes as well. While most of these pipes have been phased out, they're still in use, as we've come to find out from Flint.) Lead was banned from paint in 1978 and the US Environmental Protection Agency phased out lead from gasoline in 1996, but by that point, the amount of lead in the environment was overwhelming, with chronic lung conditions already at the forefront of health issues.

As more factories developed, more pollution, minus any regulations, was released into the air and water. These pollutants were also being deposited into the soil through the air and through toxic rain (rain polluted by high amounts of chemicals in the atmosphere). We started to have, for the first time ever, a buildup of toxins and pollutants in the soil for future generations.

As we evolved and modernized even more, particularly after World War II, our environment became even more toxic. Cigarettes were mass produced, becoming popular and adding to the air pollution (indoors and out) and to the developing health crisis. DDT, or dichlorodiphenyltrichloroethane, was used during World War II to control diseases like lice-borne typhus and mosquito-borne malaria. Once the war was over, DDT was used during aerial spraying as a way to control mosquitos in communities. Farmers also used chemical herbicides and pesticides—many of which, like DDT, got their successful start during WWII—to control weeds and insects and raise their crop yield. The majority of these biocides had delayed effects on human health, with one of these effects being cancer.[16] This is still true today.

• **Chemicals in Our Food Supply** After World War II, the focus was on producing more food (particularly convenience foods) for more people. With so many women having left the home during the war to work, there wasn't as much societal pressure for women to stay at home once the war had ended. Now there were often two parents working outside the house, so the emphasis shifted from nutritious whole foods grown in the backyard garden to foods that could be prepared quickly in the microwave, which was introduced in 1946. Spam, a mix of processed pork and other ingredients including the preservative sodium nitrate, was introduced in 1937, summing up the advances in processed foods at this time.[17] What's more, the first McDonald's, the king of convenience foods, opened in 1955. Portion sizes started increasing after the 1950s too, so not only were more people eating processed foods devoid of necessary nutrition, they were eating more of it.

Food itself was becoming littered with chemical ingredients that one couldn't pronounce in order to make processed food more palatable and shelf stable so it could last longer. Coloring additives and enhancers for texture, flavor, and aroma were also added. In fact, the 1960s has been called the "heyday of artificial flavors."[18] Processed food that didn't need refrigeration also negated the need for food-preserving bacteria (the early probiotics); in refrigerated foods, citric acid and other stabilizers were added as preservatives. The result: we became less likely to eat a daily supply of healthy bacteria in our diets to protect our guts.

A little-publicized change in the food supply also happened over the latter half of the twentieth century. Iodine, a trace mineral critical for the production of the thyroid hormones that control metabolism, body temperature, and proper growth and development (including muscle development), was replaced in breads with potassium bromate.[19] Iodine or iodate (iodized salt) was considered a bread conditioner; it made breads palatable—that is, until potassium bromate (or bromated flour) was discovered and put into the food supply. Potassium bromate was found to make bread fluffier and softer like the bread so many of us are used to eating today. Gone was the grainy brown bread of the previous era. While some bread companies have gotten rid of potassium bromide in their bread products today, many nonorganic bread products still contain this chemical. (Bromine chemicals were also added to mattresses, carpets, and clothing as a flame retardant.) The problem with bromines and other halogenated compounds, as these chemicals are often called, such as fluorine (found in fluoride) and chlorine (found in our water supply, as well as in swimming pools and hot tubs), is that they compete for iodine binding sites in the body. This means that all cells dependent on iodine for healthy function, including those of the breasts, ovaries, uterus, and prostate, then become disrupted by the lack of iodine and the subsequent absorption of these compounds. That's why bromine, fluorine, and chlorine are considered "endocrine disruptors." They disrupt the endocrine system by not allowing for the production of optimal hormone levels by the thyroid gland, the breasts, the ovaries, the uterus, and the prostate gland.

Other common sources of halogens today include plastic food containers (many of which contain bromine), citrus-flavored sodas (which contain brominated vegetable oils), nonorganic produce sprayed with pesticides and herbicides that contain bromine chemicals (one culprit: nonorganic strawberries, which are often sprayed with methyl bromide, a toxic pesticide, when they are starter plants in nurseries), toothpastes and mouthwashes that contain fluoride, some hair dyes in the form of sodium bromate, and even some cosmetics as the preservative benzalkonium.

As iodine consumption dropped 50 percent since the 1970s, is it any wonder then that iodine deficiency has increased? Some experts believe that the rate of iodine decrease parallels the increasing rates of endocrine cancers, particularly breast and prostate, which have consistently been on the rise since then.[20]

THE BODY AS OUR GUIDE

It was the Greek physician Hippocrates who, back in 400 BC, made observation of a patient and reasoning about the source of illness a critical part of medical care. The idea behind this, Hippocrates believed, was that observing a patient's outward signs was key to discovering what was ailing that person and vital to getting that person well again. As he said in one of the many medical books he wrote, *On Forecasting Diseases*:

> First of all, the doctor should look at the patient's face. If he looks his usual self this is a good sign. If not, however, the following are bad signs: sharp nose, hollow eyes, cold ears, dry skin on the forehead, strange face colour such as green, black, red or lead coloured. If the face is like this at the beginning of the illness, the doctor must ask the patient if he has lost sleep, or had "diarrhoea," or not eaten.[21]

This is similar to the clinical observation we use in medicine today, minus a vital Hippocratic aspect: a holistic observation of *all* aspects of a patient, from how they look to how they're sleeping and eating to how they're going about living their daily lives to the environment (home and office) they're spending their days in.

Think about the last time you visited a doctor to discuss an illness or something bothering you: a lingering cough, a rash on your arm, a persistent lack of energy, sporadic bloating or gas, or an inability to get a good night's sleep (to name just a few of the symptoms plaguing so many Americans). Whatever the problem, the visit probably lasted ten minutes, maybe less. Your blood pressure was checked, your heart rate and rhythm were checked, your ears were examined, as was your throat, and your lymph nodes were prodded. Possibly even a reflex "hammer" was used to check the reflexes of your tendons. These outward clinical signs are important as one part of a medical diagnosis, but they are not the be-all and end-all when it comes to diagnosing an illness or disease.

You most likely went home with a prescription drug to treat the symptoms: a cough medicine, a cortisone cream, a sleeping pill, or possibly an antidepressant. And then, once the symptoms were gone, a different problem/symptom gradually developed, seemingly separate but sourced from the same causal issue.

While these prescription drugs can and do clear up the symptoms, as I've discussed, they haven't actually solved the underlying problem. Today, unlike fifty years ago, there is also likely not merely one health problem triggering the symptoms, which is why a singular "fix" can't work to heal patients.

We're now at a point in our medical evolution where we must progress again for the sake of our health. And, as with all major evolutionary events, we must change in order to make it happen. We need to tap into the history of our medical evolution and go back to listening to all aspects of the body as Hippocrates and so many of the earliest healers recommended, tuning in to what our bodies are telling us. Yes, we should continue to use the incredible medical therapies and treatments available today to deal with "acute medicine." This includes prescription medicine that has saved millions of lives and given back life to those whose lives were unlivable without it. But we need a solution for *long-term* "wellness." We need answers to the questions: How do we regain balance and health once chronic illness has set in? And how do we prevent chronic disease from developing in the first place?

In order to understand what makes us sick, we must first define what makes us well. By defining the tenets of health and wellness, we can then begin to understand what's wrong when disease sets in. Only in this way can we understand how to reclaim our health and once again become A Nation of Well.

PART II

What Does It Mean to Be Healthy?

*Nobody can be in good health if he does not have all the
time fresh air, sunshine, and good water.*

—Chief Flying Hawk

3

How Do We Stay Healthy?
Optimizing Our Inner Ecosystem

The standard textbook definition of "health" is the state of being free from illness or injury. But health goes way beyond that. Imagine the times when you did feel healthy: you had energy to do all the things you needed to do in a day, be it exercising, working, taking care of a family, engaging in a hobby, or socializing with friends, as well as performing the day-to-day mundane activities of life, like grocery shopping, carpooling, housecleaning, and gardening. You slept well, and you woke up feeling refreshed. You also had a positive can-do attitude about life, that there was really nothing you couldn't do. You were happy and experienced a sense of fulfillment. But for so many living with chronic illness and disease, day-to-day living often becomes a struggle, as does keeping a positive attitude about the future. But this state of true health, as I call it, is completely within reach. It can be yours again, if you take charge of your body and refuse to accept a disease diagnosis as a forever branding that your body isn't whole or isn't working properly and won't ever work properly anymore. Our bodies are incredibly powerful and extremely elegant. The mere fact that we have over thirty-seven billion enzymatic reactions per second, every day—building things, removing things, communicating with other cells, allowing us to see, allowing our heart to work, giving us the ability to walk and talk (to name just a few)—is enough to create a respectful pause on how awe-inspiring the body is. What is most incredible, however, is the body's amazing ability to respond to its stressors and to stabilize or heal itself. Its incredible inertia toward wellness is an evolutionarily conserved principle; without it, we would have become extinct long ago. In other words, if given the right cellular building blocks, the body will naturally heal itself. This simple truth has been forgotten in modern medicine today. We no longer respect the body for what it is trying to do for us.

Through over a decade of working with chronically ill patients, with detailed research pertaining to each case, a beautiful understanding of how exactly the body works to overcome illnesses has emerged. Understanding this natural flow of the body toward wellness is a first step on the path to optimal health. Let's start with the following analogies to better understand how our bodies work. I use these descriptions with patients when discussing their health.

- **Our Health = A Seesaw** *Our goal is to keep this seesaw strong and balanced. Genetics = the length of this seesaw.*
- **The Body = A Flow System** *Health is maintained by a natural flow system within the body.*
- **The Gut = The Body's River** *Keeping this river flowing optimally maintains our inner ecosystem and keeps our bodies in good health.*
- **The Microbiome = The Gut's Riverbed** *This is a massive biofilm that includes bacteria, fungi, and parasites, as well as all the metabolites or products of metabolism they need to survive. This is an ecosystem inside us.*
- **The Liver & Gallbladder = Our Filter & Pump** *The liver works to keep the river and riverbed clean, while the gallbladder helps to maintain the flow in the river.*

- **The Immune System = Our Riverbank Guards** *The immune system senses the quality of the river and riverbank and then, in response, creates tolerance or inflammation in the body.*
- **The Lymphatic System = Our Border Defense** *With all its tributaries, this system is an extension of the immune system guarding the periphery.*
- **The Vagus Nerve = Our Telephone System** *The vagus nerve is the parasympathetic nervous system that transmits impulses downward from the brain to the gut but also upward from the gut to the brain, a process known as "bidirectional signaling."*
- **Our Thoughts & Feelings = Our Energy Field** *Our thoughts and feelings define the energetic field that surrounds the body. Staying positive and maintaining a sense of gratitude keeps both our energy field and our cells resonating with healing frequencies.*

OUR HEALTH = A SEESAW

Going back to Hippocrates, almost all health conditions can be described from the perspective of too much of something that shouldn't be there or not enough of something that needs to be there. In other words, when illness or disease occurs, the body is simply out of balance. The best way to understand this is by comparing the body to a seesaw. When the seesaw is tipped too much in one direction, so too are we and we don't feel well. When it's tipped too far in the other direction, the same thing happens. As the seesaw begins to tip in one direction or the other, symptoms begin to manifest themselves. Mild symptoms often start without much regularity but, if ignored, as the seesaw tilts even more, the symptoms get worse and/or more frequent. We get headaches, joint pain, swelling, stomach upset, chronic fatigue, chronic rashes, insomnia, and/or experience bloating and belching. Medical experts are now beginning to understand that many of these symptoms are due to epigenetic effects on the body, which reflect all things that have been acquired by our DNA either through the birth process or after birth. The key is that epigenetic effects can be reversed. In other words, unlike genetic effects that cannot be changed, epigenetic effects can be returned to "normal." This stops the progression of a disease but cannot always repair what has happened already.

This seesaw effect, or attempt at balancing, occurs every single day within the body, often unbeknownst to us. Once symptoms start, however, we must pay attention as the struggle within the body is starting to become unmanageable. These symptoms are the body's cry for our help. Ignoring the symptoms or quieting them temporarily with medications doesn't fix the problem or cure the imbalance; it only causes them to worsen. This out-of-balance seesaw, which isn't being readjusted, then becomes the reason chronic ailments, from autoimmune disease to cancer, begin over time. To put it simply, in order for anyone to recover from their chronic condition, the body must be relieved of whatever is making that person's particular seesaw tip too far in either direction. I call these things that tip our seesaws "stressors" on the body (see page 95).

Optimal health, what it is and what it takes to achieve it, is constantly fluctuating based on the stressors taking their toll on your body at any given moment, along with the "balancers," as I call them, that you have in your body at that time (read more about this in Chapter 4). These balancers help outweigh the stressors and keep your seesaw in balance and you healthy. In other words, there's a health tug-of-war going on within our bodies every minute of every day. The more balancers you have in your body each day to outweigh the stressors, the healthier you'll be and the less chance you'll be afflicted by illness, chronic ailments, and disease.

The length and strength of each person's bodily seesaw is dependent on genetics. In other words, there are people who have stalwart constitutions whose health is harder to throw off balance. This is the person you know who doesn't eat particularly well but never seems to get sick, despite the latest bug going around. Then there are those people who are easily thrown off balance. These patients often have a seesaw that's shorter and more likely to tip. Once we start to look at health in these terms, that each person is unique and is dealing with a different set of genetics as well as a varied set of stressors and balancers, we can begin to better understand who is getting sick and why.

THE BODY = A FLOW SYSTEM

The body naturally flows toward health. It has taken many years and hundreds of patients' recoveries to see this firsthand. In order to understand this concept further and appreciate how the body truly works, we must visualize our health in three dimensions. One way to do so is to picture the body having a large river on the inside called the gut. Lining this river is the microbiome or riverbed. The filter that keeps this river and riverbed clean is the liver, and the pump that keeps the river flowing throughout the body is the gallbladder.

Now continue to visualize this river and riverbed as I describe how the body works. We take in nourishment (as well as toxins) in the form of food and water or other liquids and substances. Some enter the body through the mouth, but others enter through the skin or other mucous membranes like the nose. These substances make up our "river." Once inside the body, in a filter-like action, the liver determines whether the substance is something to absorb and utilize or something to detoxify. If it's a nutrient, it gets absorbed. If it's a toxin, it gets detoxified by the liver or stored in that sponge-like area outside of the cells called the extracellular matrix. Once stored in the extracellular matrix, a toxin can remain indefinitely, or worse, if the matrix can no longer hold it because the concentration is too great, the toxin passes into cells where it can potentially affect our DNA.

While the liver should technically be able to filter all the toxins the body takes in, it's unable to today. Because of the amount of toxins we're being exposed to, the liver simply cannot detoxify all these toxins "on the spot," which means more and more toxins are building up in our extracellular matrix and subsequently making their way into our cells. Once inside our cells, these toxins begin to influence our genetics (an epigenetic effect).

When working optimally, with an efficient "pump" system (the gallbladder), the flow system within our body is a lot like the rhythm of waves. Toxins flow in and flow out like waves roll toward the shore and then recede. The trouble begins when the "pump" isn't working efficiently and these toxins flow in and can't flow out. Once this happens, the body must be helped to detoxify or filter, since toxins stuck inside the cells or extracellular matrix may never spontaneously release. Visualize this like debris in the water that rides in on a big wave and gets trapped on the shore instead of flowing back into the water with the next wave.

Like this debris stuck high up on the shore, these toxins can remain in the cell indefinitely unless the "pump" or gallbladder is jump-started, the water begins to flow again, and the process of detoxification or filtration in the liver is intentionally encouraged. This is where I start with all of my patients, assessing their toxicity and determining the most successful strategy for aiding detoxification. There are multiple forms of detoxification that can help. These include oral detoxification, intravenous or IV detoxification, sweat through sauna, fasting, and colonics (see page 67). All these methods create a wicking action within the body that helps draw toxins out of the cell and extracellular matrix, through the liver, and into the waste matter of the body, eventually exiting the body as sweat, urine, or feces.

This wicking process is similar to cleaning a house. If you want to clean out the bedrooms (i.e., the cells and the extracellular matrix), you must first open up the doors, hallways, and stairwells (i.e., the gut and the microbiome) so the toxins can exit. Then if you apply vacuum pressure to the house (i.e., through the pump system or gallbladder), all the dirt in the bedrooms is likely to come out. This is the same concept that governs detoxification and the body's natural flow systems. Harnessing this flow system is critical to recovering from chronic illness. This is why, when a patient talks about symptoms of chronic constipation or "never sweating," it's particularly concerning to me. In these cases, the flow system has shut off and we must get it restarted in order to help rid the body of toxins and return it to optimal wellness. Once we begin to visualize how our bodies take part in this flow toward balance and wellness, health begins to make more sense.

THE GUT = THE BODY'S RIVER

The gut is where our health begins. This long tube, which begins in the nose and mouth and continues through to the anus, encompasses the mouth, esophagus, stomach, and the small and large intestines.

The gut or "river" begins its work when you eat. Enzyme-rich saliva is produced when you chew, breaking down food so it can be moved to the gut through the esophagus, the muscular tube between the mouth and the stomach. Because saliva contains antimicrobial substances, it aids the immune system and the body in staying healthy by being a first line of defense against harmful bacteria entering the body through the mouth.

Once in the stomach, gastric juices further break down food, extracting key nutrients. Some of these nutrients are transported into the body through the bloodstream, but most are absorbed into the body after the food passes through to the small intestine. It's here that food is mixed with bile, which is produced by the liver and released from the gallbladder, and pancreatic enzymes from the pancreas. The bile helps to further break down food, particularly fats, into substances the cells can utilize. Cells lining the small intestine also produce intestinal juices that aid with the digestion of food. Nutrients from food are then absorbed into the bloodstream through villi, tiny finger-like structures with blood vessels in the lining of the small intestine. The remainder of the food moves to the large intestine, which is lined with bacteria to help further digest it. Anything that can't be digested or used by the body is excreted through the feces. This includes waste from cells and germs. Understanding the digestive process is essential to appreciating a critical part of our health: the body's microbiome.

THE MICROBIOME = THE GUT'S RIVERBED

The term "microbiome" was coined in 2007 during the Human Microbiome Project (see next page), the formal study of the microbiome by the National Institutes of Health. This microbiome is an internal ecosystem that includes bacteria, fungi, and parasites, and all the metabolites or products of metabolism they need to survive. The gut is often referred to as the microbiome because it contains nearly thirty-five trillion bacteria, at least ten bacteria for every human cell. In fact, it's estimated that the bacteria in our bodies on average weigh up to six pounds, and in some people, up to twelve pounds![22] The microbiome is also home to fungi and parasites living with bacteria in a mutually beneficial environment. Any imbalance in the microbiome (referred to as dysbiosis), which can be bacterial, fungal, and/or parasitic, is the root today of almost all chronic inflammation and the beginning of almost all chronic ailments.

It's the number and diversity of these microorganisms in our intestines that we are coming to discover is the critical link to better health. This internal ecosystem regulates inflammation, defines our immunity, prevents allergies, and helps to detoxify us.

THE HUMAN MICROBIOME PROJECT

The formal study of the microbiome began in this country under the auspices of the National Institutes of Health Human Microbiome Project. With the advent of a new biochemical testing method called "shotgun sequencing," we were able to isolate DNA from single cells rather than culturing stool, which until then had been the only reliable method available to us. In other words, before the project began, we knew only that stool had certain bacteria that grew in a petri dish when cultured. With this new sequencing technique, we were now able to isolate DNA from single cells, and we found that stool had not hundreds of different strains but *thousands* of potential strains of bacteria not yet discovered. This is how our knowledge of infection (and bacteria in the body) went from a few hundred strains of bacteria to over ten thousand in nearly five years. (If you ever wonder why gut health, and the use of probiotics, seemed to grow out of nowhere, this is how it all started.) A staggering change in medicine dawned when we realized the complexity of our gut and that we are not sterile but instead living in balance with trillions of microbes every minute.

At the time the project was launched, we knew of somewhere between two hundred and three hundred potentially infective bacteria that could invade our bodies. Today, that number is over fourteen thousand and growing. This is a dramatic shift in how we view our health. We are hosting trillions of bacteria all the time, including thousands of different strains, both bad and good. So why are we not sick? If there is a balance of good and bad bacteria in the gut (think of the seesaw analogy), we don't get sick. But when we start to lose this balancing act (i.e., the harmful bacteria begin to flourish over the beneficial bacteria), we become ill.

Also emerging is the discovery of the incredible fungal community within our gut or "*myco*biome," a term that was coined in 2010. Since then, groundbreaking research is beginning to look at the fungal community that lives in the body. Numerous research articles have been published on the powerful role that fungi in our gastrointestinal tract play in terms of our health.[23] This mycobiome is part of our global microbiome, but it has a regulatory effect on health that we're realizing could be ten times as powerful as that of the microbiome or bacterial element.

The microbiome is essentially a large biofilm (see next page) that lines our gut cells or enterocytes. A biofilm in nature can be seen as the slimy layer on a rock on a river's edge. This "slime" represents bacteria, fungi, and parasites that inhabit the water of the river and have made their way to the rock's edge to survive. The organisms themselves produce the slime or extracellular polymeric substance (EPS) to protect themselves. This way, the water of the river does not wash them away. This very same phenomenon is what begins in our gut immediately after birth, when our microbiome begins to form. This large biofilm begins in our nose and extends throughout our intestinal tract, all the way down to our anus. It's within this layer that the bacteria, fungi, and parasites reside, all offering metabolic byproducts to one another to allow for their survival. Once they attach themselves to the inside of the gut, it's the slimy EPS or biofilm that protects the microbes, preventing the bacteria, fungi, and parasites from being easily released into the stool.

WHAT ARE BIOFILMS?

Biofilms don't exist only in the gut; they're found everywhere in nature. They are essentially a collection of bacterial, fungal, and/or parasitic cells that stick together and onto surfaces in our bodies (for example, within the gut and also on our teeth, as plaque) and in our environment (such as on a rock near the water's edge). Another example is the sticky ring on a glass of water that's been left for days without cleaning. It represents the microbes that ended up in the water, or were already present in the water itself and/or the air that made their way to the glass's edge. Once there, the microbes began to produce the extracellular polymeric substance or EPS. When bacteria stick to a surface, they produce this EPS that both feeds and protects them, which may be why biofilms have been regularly referred to as "cities for microbes."

Biofilms won't simply disappear when the water in the glass is emptied or the rock is removed from the water's edge. They need to be actively scrubbed off since they are "stuck." This is the defensive mechanism of microbes to ensure their survival. They're that resilient. Having evolved from nature, it makes perfect sense, then, that the microbes' way of surviving harsh conditions likewise occurs inside our bodies.

These biofilms, however, can protect both good *and* bad bacteria, making them harmful or beneficial to us depending on the balance of the bacteria being hosted. It's through these biofilms that harmful bacteria can evade the immune system and even antibiotics, which is what happens with long-term infections that have gone undiagnosed and untreated in the body, making them harder, though not impossible, to treat.

Most chronic diseases today involve low-grade infections (either bacterial, fungal, parasitic, or all three) that are contributing to the ongoing symptoms. To address these infections successfully, we must also address the biofilms they live in.

Every Body's Microbiome Is Unique

Our individual microbiome is defined by various factors, including how we were delivered at birth, what area of the country we live in, our diet, our medication usage, and even our age. Let's look at these influences on the microbiome more closely.

• **It all begins at birth.** One of the reasons I ask all my new patients how they were delivered, via vaginal birth or via C-section, is because babies begin the development of their microbiome starting at birth. Part of the microbiome is inherited from our mothers, from both her intestine and her vagina if it's a vaginal birth. In fact, there is research that points to vaginal births helping to properly colonize an infant's gastrointestinal tract with bacteria from the mother's vagina, as compared with a C-section. As a baby passes through the vaginal canal, the mouth of the baby is colonized with the mother's vaginal bacteria, which then begin populating the baby's gut. If the mother is healthy and has a robust balance of bacteria in the gut, the bacteria she carries in her vagina are ideal for a baby's healthy immune system. Babies born via C-section haven't had this opportunity to populate the gut with a mother's vaginal bacteria—until now. In a small pilot study, researchers exposed babies born via C-section to their mother's vaginal secretions within the first two minutes of birth. Their goal was to help recreate the natural transfer of bacteria from the birth canal to help seed a baby's microbiome. The results are fascinating. The researchers were able to partially restore vaginal microbes in C-section babies.[24]

But what happens if a pregnant mother has had vaginal or gut-related issues (e.g., chronic yeast infections or other bacterial infections)? In these situations, it's common for this dysbiotic bacteria to be transferred to a baby via vaginal secretions, resulting in conditions like colic. In these situations, the bacteria the babies receive may not be ideal for their early tummies and may cause them cramping and other discomforts. This is an area where our current approach could easily shift to help our infants.

Prescribing babies with colic a probiotic designed for infants can prevent many nights of crying and fussiness. At this age, simple changes in gut ecology can stave off colic, chronic ear infections, eczema, and even asthma, all of which are conditions that reflect a disturbed microbiome in babies and young children. I have seen this time and time again in my clinic, particularly with one of my youngest patients, three-month-old Toby.

When Toby's mom brought him to see me, he was covered in eczema and had perpetual colic, never sleeping for more than twenty minutes at a time. He was exhausted and so was his mom. After examining Toby, I decided to first do a stool test to determine what was out of balance. My reason for doing this: the skin is a secondary organ of detoxification in the body and, in particular, for the gut. In other words, when there is a microbial imbalance or dysbiosis that exists within the body, and more specifically within the microbiome, it causes chronic inflammation. When the body is struggling to manage this inflammation, it will often evidence first in bowel patterns and second in the skin. It stood to reason then that a stool test might tell us what we needed to know to help Toby with his eczema. The results were as I expected. Toby had a mixture of dysbiotic bacteria in his stool, indicating that a microbiome imbalance was triggering his eczema and colic. While Toby had been delivered vaginally, his mother was an ICU nurse who regularly worked with patients who had bacterial infections. Through her work while she was pregnant, her skin had picked up bacteria and, while she did not get sick from the bacteria, they had been transferred to Toby and were too much for his immature digestive system to handle.

Dysbiosis is extremely common today and manifests not only as eczema and colic in infants but also as irritable bowel syndrome, inflammatory bowel disease, bacterial vaginosis, acne, chronic sinusitis, asthma, allergies, and more in both adults and children. When dysbiosis is identified and treated, the symptoms go away, sometimes quite readily. Sadly, though, when this condition is present during pregnancy, the baby inherits the same bacteria the mother has and the cycle is simply perpetuated. Dysbiosis is one of the most common causes of colic and infantile eczema today. If identified early, it's easy to fix and spares a baby many months of discomfort and/or progression to more serious conditions like chronic ear infections and/or asthma.

Dysbiosis is one of the most common causes of colic and infantile eczema today. If identified early, it's easy to fix and spares a baby many months of discomfort and/or progression to more serious conditions like chronic ear infections and/or asthma.

In Toby's case, I prescribed him a specially formulated daily tea to help get rid of the bad bacteria. His mother gave him a mere teaspoon of the tea every day in a syringe or in a bottle, along with an infant probiotic. The eczema quickly went away, and Toby was back to being a happy, well-adjusted baby within only two months. When I saw him next, he was sleeping through the night and was smooth-skinned and smiling.

Toby's case was easy, but it has taken me years of experience to understand how to diagnose and effectively treat problems like Toby's. Think of how many children and adults could be treated similarly before their condition gets worse. But instead, the typical treatment might be a steroid cream to treat the eczema, which would temporarily clear it up until it flared back up worse than ever, along with other conditions like chronic ear infections and/or swollen tonsils or adenoids. Toby's case was not hard to treat, but it requires a shift in how we look at the body and what it's trying to tell us when it's unwell.

The health of an infant's gut is critical to long-term health. Studies have shown that by the age of three, the bacterial milieu of the newly formed microbiome or gut is what we take with us into adulthood. (Changing where we live, how we eat, and the medications we take will affect these bacteria counts, but the underlying populations will still be there from infancy.) As the infant's gut develops, so too does the brain. If the gut is healthy, it sends signals up to the brain allowing for optimal neuronal development and circuitry. But if an infant has had many infections in early infancy that have been treated with antibiotics, this can wipe out both bad and good bacteria in the gut, and it can negatively impact neuronal health and development. The relationship between the gut and the brain is a powerful one and is referred to as the "gut-brain axis" (more on this later when we discuss the vagus nerve on page 77).

This is why an infant's diet is so critical and why it's important to avoid medications that disturb the microbiome, if at all possible. Think of every opportunity to feed a baby or young child as an opportunity to not only help him to grow but also to nourish the gut and a growing brain.

BREAST MILK VS FORMULA? THE IMPORTANCE OF EARLY FEEDING

The health of an infant's gastrointestinal tract depends not only on a vaginal delivery but also has a great deal to do with whether an infant is fed breast milk or formula. This is another reason I always ask the question of any new patient, adult or child, whether they were breastfed or formula fed. This question often surprises my adult patients because it was something that happened so long ago and, in their minds, is seemingly unrelated to the health issue they sought me out for in the first place.

Why ask this question? Breast milk has powerful antibodies that benefit an infant and his/her gut and immune system. Scientists believe these antibodies shape lifelong immune responses. What's more, multiple medical studies have been published showing a more favorable bacterial milieu in the gut of a breastfed baby versus one who has been fed formula. This is because breast milk contains natural sugars from which gut bacteria derive energy. Molecules in breast milk made by the mother's immune system also help promote tolerance of microbes in the gut.[25]

This is why I always recommend that if moms can't or don't want to breastfeed, they should be encouraged to pump, if possible, even if they pump only small amounts of breast milk while supplementing with formula. *Any* breast milk is better than none at all, so even low milk producers are doing their babies a ton of good by offering some breast milk.

That being said, there are certain situations in which the infant cannot receive breast milk of any amount. In these situations, we are grateful for the medical advance of formula and what it offers to these babies. However, the simple addition of a probiotic in formula can go a long way to help shape the microbiome of the baby drinking that formula.

• **Our lifestyle plays a part.** Each of our microbiomes develops in tandem with our lifestyle, where we live, the environment that surrounds us, and how we live (e.g., the food we eat). An unhealthy diet filled with processed foods and lacking in enough whole foods like fruits, vegetables, whole grains, nuts, seeds, legumes, healthy fats, and organic and/or grass-fed proteins results in a lack of diversity of gut bacteria. This lack of diversity, some researchers believe, contributes to diabetes, gastrointestinal disease, and other chronic diseases.[26] Having enough different strains of bacteria in the body's microbiome is essential to health. Individuals generally have hundreds of species of bacteria within their gut though they have trillions of total microbes.

Scientists have found that diets that draw from a variety of health-promoting whole foods result in diverse gut bacteria. And what's incredible is how quickly a dietary change can affect your microbiome, within just three or four days. What this means is that you can change your diet for the better (or the worse) and start to see a difference in your health within a matter of days. What's empowering is that this is entirely in your own hands. You don't need to wait for a doctor's okay to improve your diet. For example, we know and have seen firsthand in my clinic that when a patient with asthma reduces the sugar content in his/her diet, his/her symptoms and condition improve dramatically. Scientists are now finding that this is due to something called metabolic cross talk, which is the communication or interplay between the various microbes within the microbiomes of the body. In the case of asthma, research has shown that the microbiome within the gut communicates with the microbiome in the lungs by way of the bloodstream.[27] In other words, healthy dietary changes that positively affect the gut also affect the lungs, thereby improving asthma.

• **Where we live influences our microbiome.** Our cities and towns, as well as the area of the country where we reside, affect the bacterial composition of our gut, particularly if we eat locally farmed foods. Bacteria is found in the soil of fruits and vegetables, clinging to their roots, stems, and skins. Some experts believe that eating locally helps infuse the gut with the bacteria needed to stay healthy in that particular region. But it also explains why people who live in one part of the country or world will have a completely different gut microbiome than someone who lives elsewhere.

Other factors that affect your gut microbiome are your home environment and even your office, both of which harbor their own communities of microorganisms. Many of these are tracked in from the outside and come from the skin of the people who live or work there.[28]

• **Medications affect the microbiome.** Medications, such as antibiotics, mood stabilizers, birth control pills, and steroids, can produce significant shifts in the microbiome, changing its bacterial milieu in often unfavorable ways. These shifts can have long-term consequences on our health.

Acid blockers can also be problematic long term for the gut. Since bacteria find it hard to survive in the acidity of the stomach, our bodies depend on the natural acids of the stomach as a first line of defense against infections. But acid blockers do exactly as they're named. They block the production of acid in the digestive tract to prevent conditions like GERD. In doing so, they not only trigger changes to the microbiome, they also put patients at risk for infections. While there is a place in medicine for acid blockers (I prescribe them as necessary, on a short-term basis, to those with ulcers or gastritis), there should always be a long-term plan discussed as to how to get a patient off these prescription drugs as soon as possible.

SHOULD WE BE TAKING ACID BLOCKERS FOR GERD/ULCERS?

Acid in the stomach not only helps to digest protein but also provides a natural immune barrier, since most bacteria cannot withstand the stomach's acidity. This is why acid-blocking medication, particularly when a patient is taking it long-term, can be harmful to the overall digestive process and to the microbiome.

How, then, do we deal with gastroesophageal reflux disease (GERD) or ulcers? Acid reflux, ulcers, and gastritis are major signs that the seesaw is starting to tip and the microbiome is out of balance. It turns out that most reflux is caused by inflammation in the stomach leading to *reduced* acid production, which causes food to exit the stomach too slowly and ferment instead. This rancid food is what comes back up in the form of reflux and organic acids. Yes, it is acidic, but it is not the pure hydrochloric acid that our stomach naturally produces. This acid is a mixture of stomach acid and rotten acids from partially digested food.

We have had consistent success with these clinical conditions by supplementing digestive enzymes and reducing specific inflammation-triggering foods, which can be different for everyone. Another age-old technique that often works for reflux is to use castor oil packs several times per week. This simple therapy involves applying castor oil to the skin over the area of the liver (the upper right section of the abdomen), covering it with a piece of cotton cloth (an old T-shirt will do), and placing a heating pad on top for about twenty minutes while resting. Castor oil helps to improve digestive flow through the liver. Once the forward flow improves, the reflux often resolves. Lastly, when reflux is accompanied by mild gastritis (inflammation and/or irritation of the lining of the stomach), there is a family of herbs called demulcent herbs that can be taken safely to soothe irritated tissue. These are herbs like slippery elm, comfrey, licorice, and marshmallow leaf or root. At times, I add these to a patient's protocol.

The summary here is that once again, reflux or an ulcer or gastritis are major signs that our seesaw is starting to tip and our microbiome needs to be rebalanced in order to recover optimal health. This is yet another example of how we can begin to change how we think of conditions within the context of how our bodies work.

Antibiotics are problematic for the microbiome for numerous reasons. Of course, I prescribe antibiotics when needed but only for severe infections. Many times, antibiotics are prescribed today for viral infections that are not resolving quickly enough when these kinds of infections, which include most upper-respiratory infections, need immune support rather than antibiotics. These antibiotics destroy both good and bad bacteria, cause yeast overgrowth, and promote biofilm formation within the microbiome, creating significant shifts in our inner ecology. This is why, at the very least, I always prescribe probiotics with antibiotics, as taking a probiotic at least two hours after taking an antibiotic helps to restore the healthy bacteria in the gut so the microbiome stays in balance. In some cases, a course of antifungal herbs or medication is also needed to help minimize fungal overgrowth due to antibiotics.

 I always prescribe probiotics with antibiotics, as taking a probiotic at least two hours after taking an antibiotic helps to restore the healthy bacteria in the gut so the microbiome stays in balance.

Antibiotics also trigger fungal, or yeast, overgrowth in the body. By disturbing the delicate balance of bacteria that live in the mucosal membranes of the body, antibiotics allow fungus to overgrow. This can manifest as vaginal infections in women or thrush in both men and women. If these conditions are present, there is a significant imbalance in the microbiome and considerations should be made to control the yeast overgrowth. New research has determined that many of the chronic gastrointestinal conditions people are struggling with are, in fact, related to the balance of fungi and bacteria in the gut.[29] When either the fungi or the bacteria get out of balance, inflammation ensues. As an example, when fungi grow unchecked, the imbalance can trigger numerous conditions from recurring urinary tract infections, digestive issues, and skin infections to joint pain and chronic fatigue syndrome.

• **Toxins alter the microbiome.** The composition and numbers of bacteria in our microbiome are affected by artificial sweeteners, chemical additives, plasticizers, pesticides, herbicides, xenoestrogens (chemicals that imitate the hormone estrogen in the body, altering the normal functioning of hormones), and other environmental toxins, including heavy metals and pollution. This means that our environmental toxicity is deteriorating the health of our microbiome, as well as the health of our bodies and that of our liver, kidneys, and other detox organs. Heavy metals like lead and cadmium (which can get into the body through the inhalation of cigarette smoke), for example, have been found to directly affect both the composition and diversity of bacteria in the microbiome. There is also a whole body of medical literature being written about persistent organic pollutants, or POPs, and the adverse effect they're having on our physiology. POPs are toxic substances like PCBs or industrial byproducts, the insecticide DDT, and dioxins or cancer-causing chemicals. These are typically transported by wind and water and they don't break down over time in the environment. While many POPs like DDT are not in use today because they are so dangerous, they still persist in our environment from years of past use.[30] Many of these chemicals released into and utilized in our environment are fat soluble and are therefore stored in our fat cells.

Another chemical that's affecting our microbiome is glyphosate, which is found in the herbicide Roundup. Glyphosate disrupts the balance of beneficial gut microbes, leading to an overgrowth of pathogens and a chronic inflammatory state in the gut. The reason glyphosate is so problematic is that it's similar in structure to glycine, a critical amino acid in the body that's involved in everything from stabilizing blood sugar and the breakdown of food into energy (i.e., our metabolism) to cognitive function and the health of our bones, ligaments, and tendons. We're exposed to glyphosate in foods in numerous ways: by eating processed foods like cereals, crackers, and chips, as well as nonorganic produce and nonorganic grains like rice, wheat, oats, barley, and quinoa. (Glyphosate is sprayed as a preharvest drying agent on nonorganic wheat, oats, barley, and other crops.) We're also exposed to glyphosate from eating what are called Roundup Ready crops (e.g., genetically modified corn, soybeans, sugar beets, and canola plants) that have been engineered to survive being sprayed with Roundup. The problem is that once it's in a food, glyphosate can't be removed by washing, cooking, or freezing, and it remains stable in products for a year or more.[31]

Exposure to glyphosate allows the body to absorb high levels of glyphosate instead of glycine, disrupting critical enzymes in the body that need to bind to glycine but are instead binding to glyphosate. This triggers everything from leaky gut syndrome and joint pain to behavioral problems and weight gain. This is a highly alarming reality. What does it say that our children are absorbing a chemical of this kind into their growing bones and muscles, not to mention their developing brains and other organs? In my practice alone, I have seen exposure to this chemical contribute to chronic behavioral issues, pediatric weight gain despite an excellent diet, psychiatric illness, chronic pain, inflammation of the tendons, and more.

Before I knew of this reality, I often wondered why parents today who are fit and healthy could have children who are overweight. This is not something that we readily saw twenty years ago. Yet today, many if not most children have soft, bloated abdomens and mid-abdominal weight gain at a young age. In fact, the obesity epidemic is affecting our pediatric population more significantly than any other. (About 13.7 million children, adolescents, and teens in the United States are obese.[32]) Are we stopping as a nation to consider why? Yes, inactivity can contribute to weight gain, but a whole other side of the equation needs to be further explored. These children are being regularly exposed to glyphosate through nonorganic and genetically modified foods and even by running barefoot through lawns that have been treated with Roundup.

• **Aging influences the microbiome.** Numerous changes occur in the gastrointestinal tract of the elderly, which can affect their microbiome. Not only do eating habits become unhealthier (resulting from changes in taste, loss of teeth, and swallowing difficulties), there's also a decreased absorption of key nutrients like calcium, iron, and B_{12}, which causes nutritional imbalances in the body. Adding to this is chronic constipation and a slowing of the digestive process, which can trigger bacterial fermentation in the gut and a shift in the bacteria present in the gut. Multiple studies have shown a shift in the microbiome of the elderly toward more unhealthy bacteria. These changes cause a decreased functionality in the gut microflora of aging adults, which can trigger decreased immunity and susceptibility to disease. As physicians, we should be questioning how much of the aging process is in fact due to this phenomenon. If we were to actively take probiotics throughout adulthood and old age, would it help prevent some of the conditions of the elderly? [33]

• **Stress shapes the microbiome.** It's well known that long-term stress contributes to illness and diseases, such as irritable bowel syndrome (IBS) and inflammatory bowel disease. One reason is that stress physically and chemically changes the makeup of our microbiome, lowering the composition, diversity, and numbers of gut microorganisms and, in multiple cases, increasing levels of fungus and triggering an imbalance in the microbiome. Research has found that this change in the microbiome in turn affects immune function, which may be why stress contributes to illness and, long term, to chronic disease. But what's interesting to note is that it also works the opposite way, where an imbalance of microorganisms in the gut can trigger stress-related conditions like anxiety and depression. So, stress triggers acute *and* chronic health conditions, but a microbiome out of balance also triggers stress. There's simply no question that getting a handle on stress will contribute quite a bit to achieving optimal health. [34]

While in many ways we are more sophisticated today as a population, these same advances—which allow us to juggle much more in our lives, creating quite a bit of stress in the process—are negatively impacting the simple bacteria inside us and creating an uphill battle in maintaining optimal wellness. The magnitude of our health crisis makes more sense when we start thinking in these terms. It is not impossible, however, to keep our guts functioning well. With a simple understanding of what does and does not impact us, and how, we can all get a clearer sense of how to stay well and recover from being unwell.

Our Microbiome Helps to Define Our Metabolism

When we don't eat for hours, our gut bacteria offer our bodies a continuous supply of vitamins and minerals through their metabolic byproducts, keeping us regular and healthy. Think about this. These trillions of bacteria living inside us are giving us all the nutrients we need to get through our day using their own metabolism. In fact, there are several vitamins for which we are entirely dependent on our gut microbes for production: vitamin K, a cofactor in clotting, as well as some of the B vitamins. Throughout the process of digestion, the intestinal florae are fermenting indigestible carbohydrates or dietary fiber and providing us with short-chain fatty acids, an important fuel source for our bodies. In this way, our gut is able to provide us with needed nutrients between periods of non-eating.

The actual types of bacteria present in our gut are associated with our weight too. For example, I have had patients tell me they haven't been able to lose weight after taking a particular medication. This is because medications, particularly antibiotics, change the microflora in such a way to lower metabolic rate or the number of calories your body burns at rest. This is why patients may in fact suffer weight gain or even loss after taking certain medicines. One study of twins and mice introduced this phenomenon. Thin mice that had been transplanted with the microbiome from an obese twin began to gain weight without a change in diet.[35] This is likely why we begin to resemble the weight pattern of our parents, since much of the microbiome is conserved from generation to generation. Imagine this and the implications it has on our obesity epidemic. Instead of drastic diets or surgery, looking to gut health may be a key first step in weight loss.

Our Microbiome Keeps Us Free from Illness and Allergies

Research is showing that gut microflora plays a key role in immune function. Not only are 70 percent of our immune cells found in our gut, but these gut microflorae also produce antimicrobial compounds called antimicrobial peptides (or AMPs) that help to fight bacteria, fungi, viruses, infections, and even tumor cells. These antimicrobial peptides are part of the natural defense system of most living organisms against invading pathogens. As such, these compounds also seem to stimulate the immune system, which aids in its perpetual fight to stay healthy. [36]

I've also found that a healthy, balanced gut seems to tremendously help those who have allergies. An imbalance of intestinal microbiota, particularly from an early age, has been implicated in the overreaction to antigens (a substance in the body that produces an immune response) and the development of allergies, asthma, and eczema.[37]

FAST FACT

I've also found that a healthy, balanced gut seems to tremendously help those who have allergies. An imbalance of intestinal microbiota, particularly from an early age, has been implicated in the overreaction to antigens (a substance in the body that produces an immune response) and the development of allergies, asthma, and eczema.

Think about this. The number of allergies, particularly in children, is on the rise. Allergies are estimated to affect up to 30 percent of adults and as many as 40 percent of children, with that number increasing every year. Allergic disease, including asthma, is the sixth leading cause of chronic illness in the United States in people of all ages. In light of these statistics, we need to start incorporating our vast knowledge of the microbiome into how we manage these conditions. This includes dietary changes that can affect the microbiome, such as reducing sugar and carbohydrates, which has been shown to help improve outcomes of allergic disease. While medicine can be lifesaving and should always be used in acute settings, recovering the body to optimal wellness should be everyone's goal for a long-term solution. Accepting allergies or autoimmune disease as permanent and managing them with long-term medications only keeps our seesaw chronically tipped, and over time the body will go on to develop more imbalance. In other words, these conditions reflect a system that's out of balance and we need to get it back into balance in order to be healthy again. In my clinic, we have treated hundreds of cases of asthma and allergies with success by simply regulating the microbiome.[38]

THE LIVER & GALLBLADDER = OUR FILTER & PUMP

If the gut can be likened to a waterway and the microbiome the riverbed, the liver (one of the largest organs in the body) and the gallbladder (a small organ within the liver) together are the filter and pump that keep things clean and flowing.

I often use a fish tank analogy with my patients to describe how this all works together in the body. When you're cleaning out a fish tank, you get rid of the gunk that's clogging up the gravel or riverbed (flush out the microbiome), you put in fresh water (eat a whole food diet and drink clean water), you clear the filter (help detox the liver), and then you turn the pump back on (stimulate the gallbladder).

As a "filter," the liver processes all things we come into contact with, both good and bad. This includes toxins, food, hormones, and medications. In fact, everything that enters the body must be filtered or detoxified by our liver, which converts toxic substances into harmless ones the body can then get rid of. If there are too many toxins, the liver is unable to immediately detoxify them and they're stored in the sponge-like area outside of cells called the extracellular matrix, flowing back to the liver if and when it is able to address them.

As a "pump," the gallbladder is essential for the regular flow of the digestive enzyme bile, which the liver produces and the gallbladder concentrates and stores for use during meals. After eating a meal, the small intestine sends a signal to the gallbladder to release bile to help break down food—specifically fats—into substances the body can use. The gallbladder kicks into action, contracting and squeezing out stored bile into the small intestine in a pump-like action. Most of the bile is then recirculated to the liver through the blood, a process called enterohepatic circulation. (It's estimated that only about 5 percent of bile is lost through this process and excreted out of the body, giving our stool its brownish color.[39]) In its optimal state, this circulation happens at least eight times per day. It's this constant production and flow of bile that helps to establish a healthy, balanced gut or microbiome.

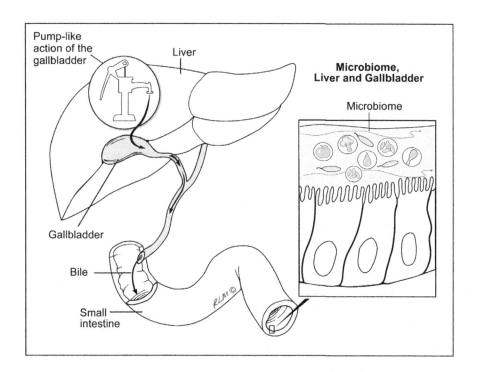

In an ideal world, the liver, gallbladder, and microbiome would all be working optimally. But in today's modern society, this is simply not the case. Not only are our diets chock-full of processed foods laden with unhealthy fats, chemical preservatives, and additives, there is also overuse of gut-altering antibiotics and medications, as well as our bodies being bombarded with toxins from all around us in our environment. Our bodies, and more specifically our liver, gallbladder, and microbiome, desperately need help. Jump-starting the liver and the gallbladder to help flush the microbiome with bile and get the enterohepatic circulation flowing optimally again is a necessary and critical step for health today.

Patrick's Story

A young patient of mine, Patrick had developed mysterious recent-onset headaches that had forced him to miss weeks of school. He had been diagnosed by several neurologists with intractable occipital neuralgia, a condition characterized by chronic pain in the upper back, back of the head, and behind the eyes. The medication that had been prescribed to Patrick wasn't helping. Since I had worked with Patrick in the past, his mom brought him back to see if I could help. While talking to Patrick and his mother, she mentioned to me that Patrick had been having nausea in the months leading up to his headaches. This was a seemingly unrelated symptom that was actually at the heart of what was wrong. Another important clue about what was causing Patrick's headaches was the area where Patrick's headaches were occurring. They were centered on the occipital ridge, the region at the back of the head where the base of the skull meets the spine. This area is on the gallbladder meridian, according to Traditional Chinese Medicine, and therefore any pain on the occipital ridge suggests that the underlying organ system, the gallbladder, is stressed. (More about Traditional Chinese Medicine later in this chapter.) In Patrick's case, his early nausea was confirmation of his gallbladder being out of balance. (Unexplained nausea is a common sign of gallbladder problems.) The key, therefore, to resolving Patrick's headaches was to give him herbal gallbladder support.

I asked Patrick's mother to give him one teaspoon of bitter herbs before his meals for one week to support the gallbladder, along with probiotics, while we waited for his blood work to come back. It's this blood work that would rule out certain infections that could also be the cause of his daily headaches.

When I called a week later with the blood results (which were negative), Patrick had already gone back to school. His mother said that, within days, his headaches had waned and by the seventh day he was "back to his old self." Imagine being given a label of "intractable occipital neuralgia" unresponsive to medication, when one week of bitter herbs to support the gallbladder put him back to health. This is a simple explanation of what can happen when body systems are supported instead of suppressed.

Both doctors and patients are missing the cries from our bodies that offer clear direction as to what is happening inside us. What's more, these imbalances generally subside fairly simply by cleaning up the diet, increasing our intake of clean filtered water, reducing unnecessary medications and, at times, supplementing with botanicals like the bitter herbs I prescribed to Patrick. Botanicals like this can help support the body until the stress is resolved.

The Beauty of Bile

As a digestive enzyme, bile is comprised of a mix of bile acids or salts, bilirubin (the brownish-yellow waste created by the breakdown of red blood cells in the body), phospholipids like phosphatidylcholine, and cholesterol, as well as water, body salts like potassium and sodium, and copper and other metals.

Bile is essential for the optimal digestion and absorption of nutrients and, in particular, fats. It also aids in the digestion and absorption of fat-soluble vitamins like A, D, E, and K. If you're eating a nutrient-rich diet and/or taking nutritional supplements but your bile isn't flowing properly, your cells may not be receiving enough, or any, of these nutrients. Instead, the body may be excreting them. This could be a reason you're simply not feeling well or you're coping with illness or disease despite all your healthy eating. The brain and nervous system are also highly dependent on fat to keep them healthy. Without the proper digestion and absorption of fat, neurological conditions from forgetfulness and lack of concentration to neurodegenerative diseases and dementia can result.

Bile also controls cholesterol production and distribution, and because bile is partially made from cholesterol, it's essential that cholesterol levels are not too low, as this would reduce the body's ability to produce bile. (It's important to note here that statins, the prescription medications that help lower cholesterol levels, can actually trigger too-low cholesterol levels, which can cause problems with the production of bile and contribute to a vicious cycle in the body.) In fact, bile is how cholesterol is eliminated from the body when levels get too high, which is a fascinating example of how the body, when functioning optimally, is always working to create balance. (It's estimated that about 500 mg of cholesterol are converted daily to bile acids and eliminated through bile.) Bile is also the major route for the excretion of trace metals, namely arsenic, copper, manganese, lead, mercury, selenium, silver, and zinc.[40]

Then there are bile acids, some of the most powerful antimicrobial and anti-inflammatory substances the body produces. It's these bile acids that help inhibit the growth of excessive biofilm and bacteria in the small intestine and, in turn, regulate the gut microbiome. What this means is that as one of the gut's primary antimicrobials, bile's release from the liver and gallbladder acts as a big flush to the microbiome, helping to reduce pathogenic overgrowth and keep things flowing.

I'd like you to stop and think about the beauty of this for a second. All of this is happening in our bodies without our ever being aware of it. And this all takes place optimally when the body, and more specifically, the liver, gallbladder, and microbiome, are in balance. Any imbalance can throw this process out of whack, which then has a domino effect when it comes to our health. We don't digest food properly (which could lead to bloating and/or gas), we can't properly digest fats (which are necessary for cellular energy and brain health), we're not able to absorb necessary nutrients (which our cells need to perform optimally), and we're not able to regulate cholesterol levels (which may become too high). The result is that we become more susceptible to inflammation, and hence illness and disease.

Reduced bile acid levels in the gut are associated with bacterial overgrowth and stagnation.[41] This stagnation in the microbiome produces excessive amounts of biofilm on the walls of the gut, which can become toxic over time, triggering conditions like chronic fatigue syndrome, irritable bowel syndrome, colitis, and small intestinal bacterial overgrowth (SIBO), which is the presence of excessive bacteria in the small intestine. A stagnant microbiome is also associated with severe bloating after meals and belching.

A slowing of the enterohepatic circulation can also cause chronic constipation, which is a problem for the body on many levels. When a patient comes to me and tells me they have one bowel movement per week, it strongly indicates *where* the trouble is in the body. This is a sign that the enterohepatic circulation has slowed significantly, the detoxification processes in the body have become compromised as a result, and there is invariably an overgrowth of the microbiome or a thickening of the biofilm within the gut. The good news is that this can all be fixed by optimizing liver and gallbladder function. In severe cases, colonics (see below) may be necessary to improve the flow in the system.

Whenever I evaluate *any* complex, chronic illness or even a simple condition in my patients, I always assess the functioning of the enterohepatic circulation, as it almost always plays a role.

COLONICS: WHY & WHEN THEY'RE NECESSARY

There has been quite a bit of skepticism in the medical community about colonics, which also go by the names "colonic irrigation" and "colon hydrotherapy."

To begin with, what actually is a colonic? In its most basic sense, a colonic is the use of warm water to help "flush" the colon and help the body release excrement. Regular waste removal is critical to a healthy, balanced body. And yes, while a body in balance should be able to regularly produce feces, removing waste and toxins from the body, much of what is actually released through a colonic is not fecal matter. Instead, what is being released is the stagnation that has built up on the walls of the upper bowel, slowing stool transit time and causing food to rot and ferment in the colon. This causes high levels of toxins to pass into the bloodstream, triggering further inflammation.

Colonics help the body to "dump" this layer of toxicity into the bowel and out for excretion, greatly increasing the rate of flow within the enterohepatic system. In essence, it's like giving the filter and pump a kick-start to help clear the clog in the drain so everything can flow better.

I have found colonics to be invaluable in helping my adult patients with chronic fatigue syndrome, neuropathy, fibromyalgia, chronic headaches, irritable bowel syndrome, small intestinal bacterial overgrowth (SIBO), and learning and behavioral disorders. Why? Brain health is incredibly dependent on the health of the gut (the so-called "gut–brain axis"). After having colonics, patients report more energy, clearer thinking, and an overall sense of wellness that they hadn't had before. By kick-starting enterohepatic circulation, colonics have been a critical part in returning my patients to a state of wellness.

There are two types of colonics being used today: Open System Colonics and Closed System Colonics. As a medical professional, I prefer Open System Colonics for my patients. They are inherently easier on patients, pose less risk, and are generally preferred by patients due to comfort. That being said, with the correct medical supervision, the Closed System can be just as effective. I do not, however, recommend colonics for everyone. Every patient should consult with his/her medical doctor before considering any therapy.

Bile and Phosphatidylcholine

Bile is critical for the production of a highly important fat—or phospholipid—for colonic health called phosphatidylcholine (PC). When bile makes its way down to the small intestine from the gallbladder, it stimulates the production of phosphatidylcholine, which is then secreted into the large intestine or colon. PC then washes through the large intestine and protects the colonic mucosa, or intestinal lining, from the enormous burden of bacteria within the gut. Without sufficient PC, chronic inflammation within the colon begins and, in certain cases, can lead to irritable bowel syndrome—or in more severe cases, inflammatory bowel disease like ulcerative colitis. Recovering phosphatidylcholine levels in the lower bowel, either through diet or supplementation, is often enough to reverse the inflammation and allow the flow system to continue uninterrupted.[42]

When it comes to diet, phospholipids like PC are extracted from foods such as egg yolks, liver, unpasteurized or raw dairy, and heavy cream. Practically speaking, we no longer eat enough of these foods today to be able to get adequate amounts of PC. Therefore, the natural method to rectify this is to take phosphatidylcholine supplements.

But what if someone no longer has a gallbladder to release enough bile into the small intestine, signaling for the secretion of phosphatidylcholine? This results in dwindling levels of PC over time, which can set up a patient for more colon inflammation. It's also impossible for those without a gallbladder to optimally absorb fat-soluble vitamins long term since bile is a critical part of this process. This is why, for these patients, I recommend long-term supplementation with ox bile (a purified form of bile) at mealtimes, which I have found to be safe.

The Liver and Cholesterol Production

The processing of cholesterol by the liver is a highly misunderstood concept in medicine today. Nearly 85 to 95 percent of the circulating cholesterol

TAKING THE MYSTERY OUT OF GALLSTONES

Gallstones are hardened collections of digestive fluid that build up in the gallbladder and range in size from the tiniest grain of sand to a golf ball. They can be composed of hardened cholesterol (found in bile) or bilirubin (red blood cell waste that's also part of bile). Some people experience no symptoms from gallstones, while others experience pain, particularly if a gallstone is large and blocking the flow of bile.

It's been the protocol of modern medicine to remove the gallbladder entirely when gallstones trigger symptoms like abdominal pain after meals in order to prevent a gallbladder "attack." (Continued pain in the upper right or middle of the abdomen, fever, nausea, and diarrhea are all symptoms of a gallbladder "attack.") In fact, the gallbladder is perceived as "nonessential" to our digestion. This is not true. As already noted, the gallbladder is absolutely essential to store the ever-important bile for optimal digestion and the ensuing health of the microbiome. The bigger issue with any patient is *why* the body is creating gallstones in the first place. Understanding this "why" is critical to keeping our seesaw balanced.

When I work with patients, together we begin to understand the underlying trigger(s) of the gallstones, which are stressors such as a nutrient-deficient diet and/or a microbiome imbalance. Then we develop a plan to address these triggers and restore balance to the body. What's important to recognize, however, is that the gallbladder is an extension of a larger organ, the liver. If the gallbladder is being affected by these stressors, it stands to reason that these same stressors are also negatively affecting the liver, as optimal bile flow begins with the liver. The state of the liver is something that must be addressed to get the gallbladder functioning optimally again.

in our bodies is actually produced in our liver. But we assume the reasons for an elevated cholesterol panel are the eggs we're eating for breakfast or the butter we're using on our toast. Food-borne cholesterol, however, accounts for no more than 15 percent of our total cholesterol pool, so when cholesterol is elevated, it's more appropriate to ask, *Why is my body making extra cholesterol?* instead of *What's wrong with my diet?*

> **FAST FACT**
>
> Nearly 85 to 95 percent of the circulating cholesterol in our bodies is actually produced in our liver. But we assume the reasons for an elevated cholesterol panel are the eggs we're eating for breakfast or the butter we're using on our toast. Food-borne cholesterol, however, accounts for no more than 15 percent of our total cholesterol pool, so when cholesterol is elevated, it's more appropriate to ask, *Why is my body making extra cholesterol?* instead of *What's wrong with my diet?*

There are many reasons the body makes extra cholesterol, but the most fundamental reason is a deficit of critical fat families in the body. Cholesterol defines animal life in that all animals have cholesterol in their cell membrane, whereas plants do not. This actually underscores the importance of cholesterol in the body. It is the reason we are an "animal." It is also the most common fat in the central nervous system, accounting for nearly 50 percent of the brain. In addition to cholesterol, however, we also have two other families of fats: the phospholipids I mentioned earlier and sphingomyelins, another family of fats found in dairy and eggs. Since our cell membranes require all three of these fat families to be present, when one kind of fat is low in numbers, the body will naturally make more of another to compensate. In my practice, when working with patients with elevated cholesterol, we always test the levels of the other fats in the body to determine what might be in deficit (e.g., phospholipids and/or sphingomyelins) and supplement accordingly to achieve balance. Once in balance, many patients' cholesterol levels will naturally drop by tens of points. I had one patient drop her cholesterol levels over seventy points in two months with appropriate supplementation, without changing one thing in her diet!

THE IMMUNE SYSTEM = OUR RIVERBANK GUARDS

Much like a village built next to a river would put guards on the riverbank, so too our body protects itself from invasion at the "banks" of the gut and microbiome with our immune system. In this way, the immune system is keenly positioned to sense what's going on in the body, specifically in the river and riverbed.

An expansive network of organs, tissues, and cells (most of which reside within the gut), the immune system is constantly on the watch for invaders like bacteria, fungi, and parasites that can cause illness and disease. Key immune cells called dendritic cells are critical to this process. These nerve cells are like spiders with long "arms" that extend up into the microbiome, sense what's going on, then signal the other cells of the immune system (namely white blood cells called macrophages, T cells, and B cells) when they should stay quiet and when they need to turn on, and how. One way in which the immune system communicates from cell to cell is through chemical messengers called cytokines. Cytokines are small proteins that are released from one cell and travel either to a neighboring cell or to a distant cell through the blood. These chemicals effectively send a message by stimulating the receiving cell to act. One example of this is a fever, which occurs when the hypothalamus in the brain receives a "signal" to make the body hot in response to an invading microbe.

In the case of the microbiome, when the immune system senses an imbalance through the network of dendritic cells, it sends out cytokine messages to the rest of the body, which tell it how to respond. If bacterial invaders are sensed, the immune system sends out a message to generate the kind of inflammation that makes us feel achy and sick and even depressed. If fungal invaders are sensed, the immune system sends out a stronger signal to mount high levels of inflammation, the kind that creates body pain, fibromyalgia-like symptoms, moderate to severe headaches, and neurological symptoms and anxiety, including even panic and obsessive compulsive disorder (OCD). If a parasitic invader is sensed, the immune system sends out signals to release histamines and produce mucous in order to help dislodge the parasite from the wall of the gut, lungs, or anywhere else in the body. In fact, most allergic responses are geared toward this "weep and sweep" response, as it has been called, which helps to keep the gastrointestinal and respiratory tracts free from invading parasites.

Inflammation in this context is meant as a quick response by the body designed to control the offending organism (or heal itself after an injury or repair damaged tissue) and in a healthy system should turn off quickly. Unfortunately, in today's modern world, this is no longer happening and inflammation is not turning off quickly but instead staying on for chronic periods of time. One example of this is a patient who gets a fever, spends the day in bed, and then the next day is well. This demonstrates classic inflammation that serves a beneficial purpose. In contrast, the patient who has a slight temperature increase and remains sick for several days or even weeks is an example of low-grade chronic inflammation and a less-than-optimal immune response.

Many diseases today, including heart disease, autoimmune diseases, and cancer, are due to chronic inflammation. In these cases, the body is set up to have inflammation on all the time, much like a car in drive mode that can't stop. Most of the time, our immune system sends a strong "brake" signal to the body to stop the inflammation. But with today's modern stressors on the body, this brake signal is being worn down and many of us are left with a slowly rolling car and continuing inflammation since the body isn't sending the critical stop signal. There is quite a bit of medical research exploring ways to stop inflammation today, restoring the brake signal.

Nearly all inflammation, however, begins with an unhealthy microbiome. I know from all the patients I have treated at my clinic that when a patient has a healthy, balanced microbiome, they have a strong immune system and classic inflammation instead of chronic inflammation. Many of my patients, once recovered, will tell me that, after years of not getting a fever, they once again developed a short-lived fever when they got sick with a cold. This is a good thing. Getting a fever is normal and actually means that the body, and the immune system, are working optimally. This is another reason why honoring the body is so important when we get sick and why it's important not to suppress symptoms that develop with various kinds of medicines (e.g., cold medicines or fever reducers).

Immune Regulation: How It Works

Our incredible immune system also has "guards" throughout the body as it does within the microbiome. Its goal is to keep invaders out and destroy any that do get into the body. These guards include macrophages, T cells, B cells, and other specialized immune cells that protect against invaders with special compounds that help kill off invaders, from bacteria, fungi, and parasites to viruses and even cancer cells.

The first line of defense against invaders is one of our largest organs, the skin, which contains barriers to harmful substances. While the skin can't be penetrated unless there's a cut or opening on the surface, it is also one of the first places that inflammation in the body can manifest itself, through rashes, eczema, and acne. Other systems that help protect the body from an invasion:

- **Tears, saliva, and urine** work to help force out pathogens in the environment that could potentially cause the body harm or make it sick.

- **Mucous membranes in our nose and mouth/throat** help trap viruses, bacteria, and pathogens.

- **Mucous membranes in the vagina and bladder** help protect the onslaught of bacteria and viruses that enter the body through these areas.

- **The tonsils on the back of the throat and adenoids on the roof of the mouth** are also on the first line of defense, coming into contact with viruses and bacteria almost immediately and activating the immune system. This is a reason the microbiome and immune function of children with chronically inflamed tonsils or adenoids should be explored before surgery is performed to remove them. These are critical parts of the immune system. If they are chronically inflamed, there is a reason for it.

The tonsils on the back of the throat and adenoids on the roof of the mouth are also on the first line of defense, coming into contact with viruses and bacteria almost immediately and activating the immune system. This is a reason the microbiome and immune function of children with chronically inflamed tonsils or adenoids must be explored before surgery is performed to remove them. These are critical parts of the immune system. If they are chronically inflamed, there is a reason for it.

The other key part of the immune system is the lymphatic system, which I discuss next.

THE LYMPHATIC SYSTEM = OUR BORDER DEFENSE

While the bulk of the immune system resides within the microbiome or riverbed, the tributaries within the river are our lymphatic system. The lymphatic system is comprised of tiny conduits throughout the body that circulate a clear fluid called lymph, which contains infection-fighting white blood cells or lymphocytes. The main job of the lymphatic system is to bathe all of our cells with these wonderful immune cells. It also delivers oxygen and nutrients to the cells then carries away the waste (including carbon dioxide, viruses, bacteria, and even parasites) through the lymph fluid. The blood, along with the lymph, circulates all of this healthy, balanced fluid to nourish and protect our periphery, then circulates it back to the liver to be cleansed and sent out again. Our bodies really do work in the most elegant and intricate fashion!

These tiny vessels of the lymph system also contain all sorts of powerful immune surveillance cells that are constantly circulating through our bodies to defend us from invading organisms. This is why lymph nodes, the small, bean-shaped glands throughout the body where lymph is filtered and where lymphocytes (a type of white blood cell) are created, enlarge when the body encounters and fights an infection. When this happens, the infection is drained off to the nearest node where the immune cells fight it. As it swells, it becomes tender from the inflammation of the infection. This swelling reflects a healthy immune response.

In contrast, lymph nodes that are chronically inflamed without resolution, as in the case of the child with swollen glands in their neck or adenoids, is problematic. This is a state of dysregulation and should be considered from the perspective of *What's causing it?* instead of *How can we remove the gland (e.g., tonsils and/or adenoids)?*

The Lymph System Up Close

In addition to the lymphatic capillaries, the lymph system is composed of the following:

- **Lymph nodes**, numbering five hundred to seven hundred, which are mostly found in the middle of the body. The others are situated near the abdomen, groin, and armpits, as well as in the neck. As our bodies' filtration stations, they produce and store cells that fight illness and disease; they also filter and clean the lymph fluid as it flows through the nodes. The liver works hand in hand with the lymph system to flush waste from the body.

- **The thymus gland**, situated above the heart, which is where T cells (a type of white blood cell that helps destroy infected cells) are produced.

- **The spleen**, located in the upper part of the abdomen, which manufactures white blood cells that fight infection and disease. The spleen acts as a filter helping to "purify" the blood, removing old or damaged red blood cells, as well as any bad bacteria, parasites, fungi, or viruses it finds. The spleen is also a site where immune cells and nerves interact and is the pathway by which critical information from the nervous system gets to the immune system.[43]

- **The bone marrow**, which is the sponge-like tissue inside the bones. It produces defensive white blood cells called B cells; these make antibodies that attack, neutralize, and destroy bacteria and toxins, protecting cells.

THE VAGUS NERVE = OUR TELEPHONE SYSTEM

Named from the Latin root "vagary," or wandering, the vagus nerve is the longest nerve in the body, with long branches that touch almost all of our internal organs. This nerve extends from the brain stem all the way to the lowest part of the abdomen, essentially communicating *everything* that's happening in the body, and in the gut or microbiome, to the brain.

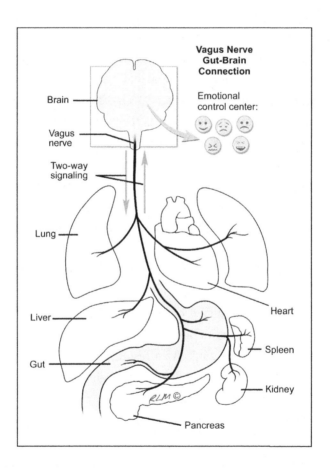

Scientists used to believe that the brain and the body were rigorously separated by what is called the "blood-brain barrier," meaning they thought the brain was protected from the blood and sheltered from much of everything else going on in the body. While the blood-brain barrier does exist to prevent the passage of harmful pathogens through the blood into the brain, it doesn't block communication with the body. In fact, just the opposite is happening. Through the vagus nerve, the brain is actually in constant communication with different organs of the body by way of a bidirectional signaling system. This allows "messages" to move constantly between the brain and the rest of the body and vice versa, which is why I refer to the vagus nerve as our internal telephone system.

The gut is central to this communication system. The brain "talks" to the gut and the gut "talks" to the brain. (This is why when we say we have a "gut feeling" about something, we're actually tapping into what our gut is telling our brain about how we should act.) This direct vagal connection from the gut to the brain is often referred to as the "gut–brain axis" and integrates what's going on in the brain and in the nervous system with what's going on in the gut.[44] In one example of this, messages leave the brain via the vagus nerve when we're hungry, signaling that we need to eat. As we eat, the stomach enlarges and an "I am full now" signal leaves the stomach and, via the vagus nerve, travels back up to the brain to tell us to stop eating. (This is one reason that eating slowly and mindfully is so important. We're giving our internal telephone system time to communicate that we're full.) The gut also sends signals up to communicate the health of the gut and microbiome to the brain, which is critical because many mental health issues from anxiety and depression to pediatric neurobehavioral issues occur when there's an imbalance in the gut.[45] As a result, physicians must start to look at gut health more rigorously in order to help their patients recover from not only mental health issues but all health problems.

The brain also corresponds with the immune system through the vagus nerve. In fact, new discoveries have revealed that the vagus nerve communicates what's happening with the spleen, the largest organ in the lymph system. The spleen can dump an army of immune cells into our system quickly when needed, to help regulate inflammation in the body.[46] When the body is relaxed and in balance, the vagus nerve communicates with the spleen saying,

Everything is okay. Your troops can rest for now. This is a superb example of the "mind–body connection" and shows how relaxation exercises like meditation and deep breathing can calm the vagus nerve, thereby helping to lower inflammation in the body.

THE VAGUS NERVE AND THE RELAXATION RESPONSE

What's fascinating about the vagus nerve is that as it extends up from the gut and down from the brain, it runs straight through the diaphragm, the "sheet" of muscles and tendons that separate the chest from the gut. When we initiate deep breathing from the diaphragm (i.e., taking slow, deep belly breaths instead of short breaths from the chest), we're actually continually massaging or stimulating this nerve. (To breathe diaphragmatically, visualize pulling in air through your toes up through your belly—pushing it out with air like a balloon—then into your chest, and then exhaling slowly. For more details on how to perform the relaxation breath, see "Your Two-Week Health-Boosting Plan," page 155.)

This stimulation of the vagus nerve has been shown to initiate what's called "the relaxation response," which in turn reduces levels of stress hormones, triggering a reduction in anxiety, anger, and hypertension.[47] In fact, some researchers have found that people who have healthy "vagal tone" (a vagus nerve that's regularly stimulated) showed a lower predisposition to stress overall, a stronger mental and physical constitution, better heart rate variability (the variation in time between heartbeats), and even better cognitive function.[48] Improved heart rate variability not only helps the health of the heart but also reduces anger, anxiety, and depression.

One theory is that when the vagus nerve is stimulated, a neurotransmitter called acetylcholine is released. It's acetylcholine that's responsible for relaxation, as well as for learning and memory. When acetylcholine is released, it signals the immune system to turn down its inflammatory response, reducing inflammation.

The Link Between Gut and Mood

You can begin to see how the gut is intricately linked to our mood and mental health. But there's more to this critical relationship. There are in fact two nervous systems within us: the central nervous system that includes the brain and spinal cord, and our enteric nervous system, which is the nervous system of our gut and represents the primordial nervous system that we evolved with. It's the enteric nervous system that lies within the tissue below the gut cells. Its complex circuitry contains over a hundred million neurons and produces over 80 percent of our neurotransmitters, including substances like serotonin, dopamine, glutamate, norepinephrine, and histamine that control our mood. This is why maintaining a healthy microbiome, which feeds the enteric nervous system, is of optimal importance in keeping our mood balanced. A healthy microbiome starts with a nutrient-rich, whole foods–based diet, not the processed foods that fill the majority of grocery store shelves today.

There is a link between the average American's diet, chock-full of these processed foods, and the depression that afflicts millions of people in our country. The lack of feel-good chemicals like serotonin that many are suffering from is due to deficiencies in the diet, which are causing an imbalanced microbiome and triggering chronic low-grade inflammation. In response, inflammatory chemical messengers, cytokines, are sent up to the brain by the immune system to initiate feelings of depression. This is why some experts are referring to depression as part of a group of symptoms in the body called "sickness behavior."[49]

In addition to the depression-like features of chronic inflammation, there is another reason why prolonged gut inflammation may cause depression. The trillions of microbes, both good and bad, within our gut depend on our intake of an essential amino acid, tryptophan, to survive. (The body can't make tryptophan. It must get it from our diet, specifically animal and plant proteins like turkey, nuts and seeds, soy-based foods, fish, and legumes.) Once it's absorbed from food, tryptophan is converted in the body to the feel-good neurotransmitter serotonin. Through evolution, our immune system devised a way to quickly lower tryptophan levels to protect us from certain kinds of invading organisms, thereby starving an invader within hours of its entrance into the microbiome. If the invading organisms remain in the body long term, however, tryptophan levels remain low and patients will ultimately start to experience a low mood and depression. When I describe this to patients, I say that there is a "trap door" that the body sends tryptophan through in order to prevent the invaders or microbes from using it to thrive. It's a very elegant system. But if this trap door stays active for weeks to months, mood is ultimately affected.

This is why scores of depressed patients on medications are unable to lift their mood long term and why the need for antidepressants is on the rise: the underlying issue (i.e., invading organisms) is not being resolved. This also explains why patients will often respond to one medication that increases serotonin levels in the body for some time but then the depression returns and the medication needs to either be increased or changed.

Checking the health of the microbiome when a patient has depression is critical, as helping to reestablish balance in the microbiome can restore the body's regular production of serotonin and recover the patient's mental health without prescription medications. I have seen this in many of my patients. As their microbiome becomes optimally balanced and they become healthy once again, they no longer need mood-stabilizing medication in order to achieve a state of happiness and joy.

THOUGHTS & FEELINGS = OUR ENERGY FIELD

When we hear about the body having an "energy field," numerous medical professionals and even patients become skeptical. But the well-known physicist Max Planck said it best: Our bodies are 99 percent energy and 1 percent matter. Yet Western medicine is largely practiced with a focus on matter and not energy. Why is this?

The most likely reason is that over time, we've been trained and conditioned to look predominately, if not exclusively, at what we can readily see, such as the body's visible systems. This is still true today despite a growing field of research launched when a compelling book, *The Body Electric,* was published in 1985. The book made a strong case for how crucial our energy field is, but whether it felt too intangible to explore or was simply too foreign to the majority of American doctors, an overarching appreciation of this invisible yet critical phenomenon never quite took hold in mainstream medicine.[50]

In a compelling examination, *The Body Electric* unveiled the fact that our bodies are not merely a collection of cells working together to keep us healthy and alive. We also produce energy and an energy field. Several health systems, such as Traditional Chinese Medicine and Ayurveda, tap into these energy fields to boost health. More specifically, these traditions believe that blockages in the energy flow within the body along energy channels or meridians translate to health problems and that unblocking this chi, or energy, helps heal the body. Researchers have even found that the body actually emits visible light, pointing to the tangible existence of this energy field, which fluctuates with our metabolic rhythms.[51]

To grasp this further, it's crucial to understand the enormous role our thoughts and feelings play in this energy field and in our health. They are a reflection of the mind–body connection we hear about all the time. Negative emotions, namely stress/anxiety, anger, cynicism, hatred, sadness, depression, and even loneliness, can put a strain on the body's energy system.[52]

FAST FACT

Negative emotions, namely stress/anxiety, anger, cynicism, hatred, sadness, depression, and even loneliness, can put a strain on the body's energy system.

We've become more aware of and focused on the toxins and chemicals in our food, water, homes, and environment around us as bodily stressors, but powerful negative emotions, which are often accompanied by shallow, stress-induced chest breaths that don't stimulate the vagus nerve, can be toxic too. Negative emotions put a stress load on the body by triggering the release of stress hormones, causing the heart to beat faster, increasing blood pressure, and even changing the heart's electrical stability, all of which, over time, can trigger inflammation and health problems like heart disease, autoimmune disease, and cancer.[53] Chronic feelings of negativity can also suppress the immune system over time, making us more susceptible to illness and disease.[54]

In one fascinating book, *The Hidden Messages in Water*, scientist Masaru Emoto found through high-speed photography that molecules of water are affected by our thoughts, words, and feelings. Emoto found that crystals formed in frozen water reveal changes with specific thoughts. More specifically, he found that "water from springs, the upper reaches of the rivers, and other natural sources creates beautiful crystals," as does water that's been exposed to loving words.[55] In contrast, polluted water or water exposed to negative thoughts forms incomplete, asymmetrical patterns with dull colors. Keeping in mind that our bodies are composed mostly of water, Emoto found, without a doubt, that the energy of positivity, love, and gratitude is powerful. It's life-changing research that carries an unmistakable message for how we should all be focusing our thoughts.

Gratitude, in particular, is essential to staying well. In fact, I've found that I have the easiest time helping patients who have a sense of gratitude in life. It seems evident that in order for the body to heal easily, positive frequency must exist within their energy field, as positive energy is necessary to rebuild and repair tissue. We can be 100 percent well and have a day that just doesn't feel right. We can also slip into focusing on the sensations of what's wrong, forgetting to appreciate all that is right. But when we take stock and appreciate all that the body is doing for us and all that the body is capable of doing, we heal faster.

Having gratitude also gives us a sense of something greater than ourselves, which often helps to reduce the negativity and stress that can overwhelm our lives. In fact, one study found that having a sense of awe and wonder in our lives, something that gratitude thrives on, not only relaxes us but has an immediate effect on our health by lowering levels of pro-inflammatory cytokines, the chemical messengers in the body.[56] It's these cytokines that can either call for the immune system to trigger inflammation in the body or let its guard down because all is well. It makes sense when you think about it. When we're filled with awe and gratitude, we're relaxed, which means the vagus nerve is sending signals throughout the body to stay calm, which in turn lowers inflammation.

If certain aspects of our lives aren't working in our favor, we must take steps, even if they're baby steps, to change them. (See the simple steps to change in "Your Two-Week Health-Boosting Plan," page 155.) It's no coincidence that when you look at the scores of people who are unhappy, anxious, or otherwise in an unhappy place, you see a rise in chronic disease. Negative thoughts simply don't make room for healing in the body. This is why I encourage patients to find at least fifteen minutes every day to do something for themselves that they love. This gives them something to look forward to and contributes to overall happiness and health.

PART III

What Does It Mean to Be Sick?

Health is not valued until sickness comes.

—Thomas Fuller

4

How Disease Takes Hold:
When the Seesaw Starts to Tip

With our bodies working actively to keep us well, what then is tipping the body's seesaw? What are the stressors causing our bodies to get off balance at an alarming rate? What is causing the rapid increase in rates of disease? These are the questions each one of us should be asking today.

Let's start with what I call "A Tale of Two Cells," one not-so-healthy from today and another much healthier from fifty years ago.

There are reasons cells were healthier fifty years ago, and it has a lot to do with our environment and what our bodies were exposed to, or more specifically, not exposed to, at the time.

A HEALTHY CELL FIFTY YEARS AGO

- **Drinking water was cleaner.** There were fewer pollutants in the water overall. What's more, The Safe Drinking Water Act was passed in 1974 and regulated the top ninety-one contaminants at the time.[57] Keep in mind that it's the cell membrane, or outermost layer of the cell, that controls what gets into the cell, including water, food, and toxins.

- **Food was healthier.** Food was made with more real ingredients and fewer processed ingredients with unrecognizable names, as well as with fewer chemical sweeteners. Bread also had less gluten in it. Today, modern varieties of bread have much more gluten, causing those with a gluten sensitivity to have even more of a reaction to it.

- **Fewer pesticides and herbicides were in use.** Biocide use ramped up after 1940.[58] Prior to that, fruits and vegetables were grown without mass-produced toxic chemicals to destroy insects, fungus, and weeds.

AN UNHEALTHY CELL TODAY

- **More chemicals are in our drinking water.** More than sixty thousand new chemicals are not regulated by the Safe Drinking Water Act. Sixty thousand! Plus, discarded prescription medications are making their way into our water supply, as are disinfectants, runoff from pesticides and herbicides from farms, and much more.[59] Our drinking water may be "legal," but it's not safe for our cells. Despite all the new chemicals in existence, not one new chemical has been added to the list of those regulated by the Safe Drinking Water Act since the year 2000.[60]

- **Food is more processed with fewer nutrients.** Food today is highly refined and contains a multitude of artificial ingredients, including sweeteners. The body is not able to recognize most of these ingredients as real food, which is putting our immune system on high alert. What's more, everything contains sugar, even simple foods like ketchup and peanut butter. Vegetable oils like canola or rapeseed oil, soybean oil, and cottonseed oil are processed oils that are high in trans fats and omega-6 fatty acids, which trigger inflammation in the body in large amounts. (Read more about the balance of omega-6 fatty acids in the body on page 134.)

- **Everything is supersized.** People are getting more of what their bodies and cells don't need, including calories and fat. This contributes to the obesity epidemic we're experiencing today. For example, soda, which is not healthy to begin with, was for decades sold in a standard serving size of twelve ounces. Today, soda is sold in "Big Gulp" sizes of sixty-four ounces.[61] In short, our cells are being inundated with junk.

- **Pesticides and herbicides are stronger than ever and more pervasive.** Insects are now becoming resistant to these chemicals, requiring more powerful biocides to be developed with even more negative effects on our bodies and our cells.

TAKING OUT THE TRASH: HOW WE STAY WELL

All cells must dispose of their waste (e.g., viruses, bacteria, parasites, germs, and damaged or superfluous material) for normal cellular functioning. This waste disposal keeps cells healthy and in balance. Now let's say your cells have fifty bags of trash to take out every single day. What you eat and drink, as well as the air you breathe and personal care products you use, affects how quickly your cells and your body are able to remove the trash. For example, if you drink one diet soda, it will take your body longer (say, six hours) to get rid of the trash. If you drink a cup of unsweetened herbal tea instead, your body is able to remove the trash in much less time. The efficiency of this critical process depends on how you treat your body. If you eat a lifetime of junk and don't take care of your body by exercising, getting enough sleep, and steering clear of alcohol, drugs, cigarettes, and toxins, your body will have a difficult time working efficiently and removing waste. Once there's a buildup of waste in the cells, the waste becomes toxic and diseases like cancer and Alzheimer's can set in.

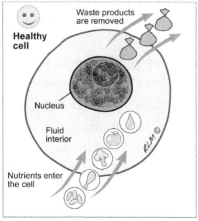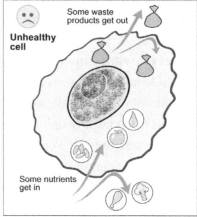

This underscores how much of your health is in your own hands, even if you're sick or have been diagnosed with a chronic disease. Everything you do affects your body, down to its most intricate cellular level. Start making small changes (See Your Two-Week Health-Boosting Plan, page 155), and your body and cells will respond accordingly in the most positive and amazing ways.

LACK OF BALANCERS: A PRECURSOR FOR DISEASE

In order to define disease today, we need to go back to Hippocrates's theory that when there is disease, there is too much of something that shouldn't be there (e.g., infection or toxin) or not enough of something that should be there (e.g., healthy bacteria, nutrients, phospholipids) or both.

Medicine as it's practiced today implies permanence to disease diagnoses, meaning once we have a chronic condition, it is unlikely we will ever be cured; the prevailing theory is that we can ease our symptoms or control progression with medication. Nowhere in this construct is the belief that true healing and a recovery to wellness can occur. But it is our job within the medical profession to understand *how* and *why*. It is my belief that almost *all* chronic conditions today can be reversed because I have seen them reversed. Most diseases today are simply a label that represents a constellation of symptoms (e.g., chronic daily headaches and fibromyalgia). These labels *can* be reversed and are often not a lifetime disorder that one must live with.

Decades ago, when we had rampant infectious diseases like tuberculosis, leprosy, flu, and syphilis, we also had plenty of balancers to outweigh the infectious stressors on our system. This meant that while a multitude of people did succumb to acute infections due to lack of effective medicines, most did not have chronic disease like so many do today. Autoimmune disease was rarely, if ever, heard of. Chronic fatigue syndrome didn't exist, nor did fibromyalgia, ADHD, autism, Asperger's syndrome, neurally mediated hypotension, dyslexia, apraxia (a motor disorder where a person cannot perform purposeful actions), and the list goes on. At this rate, experts have already predicted that chronic disease statistics will become dire.[62] Obviously, something must change or the fate of our health and our medical future is in jeopardy. A simple place to start is to examine what we need for balancers and explore why we don't have enough today.

• **Nutrient Deficiency on the Rise** The biggest issue is the lack of nutrients in our current soil. Modern farming methods and the use of powerful pesticides and herbicides have stripped nutrients from the ground, thereby stripping nutrients from the fruits and vegetables that grow in this soil. What's more, these same toxic chemicals interfere with the supply of critical nutrients to our cells. The result: our diet today is seriously lacking key nutrients like protein, vitamins like C and riboflavin (B₂), minerals like calcium, iron, and phosphorus, and healthy fats. Even if our diets were near perfect, we would have a hard time getting enough vitamins and minerals needed for optimal health from our foods. They simply no longer have enough to offer.[63]

One scientist found that nutrients were depleted from modern foods up to 38 percent.[64] Think about this. The spinach we're eating today, for example, probably contains 38 percent less riboflavin than it did fifty years ago, all because of the soil and how we're growing it. What's more, the RDA for vitamins and minerals today is what we need at the most basic level to avoid obvious signs of nutrient deficiency (e.g., to prevent conditions like scurvy from lack of vitamin C or beriberi from lack of vitamin B_1). This is not how much we need to stay optimally well. There's actually quite a difference between the RDA numbers and what our bodies need for long-term wellness.

Because we're lacking these key balancers (the nutrients the body needs in order to function at peak efficiency) in our food supply, we suffer from chronic nutrient deficiency in this country. Even worse, modern medicine doesn't test patients for nutrient deficiencies (zinc and B_6 are most common) when symptoms begin to present themselves.

And it's not only adults. The average American child's diet is deficient, particularly that of the kids who subsist on macaroni and cheese and plain pasta because that's all they want to eat. As a mother, I know that taking a hard line on food isn't easy, but we must take a hard line with our kids for the sake of their health. Children should be eating healthy, nutrient-rich foods since the goal is to feed their growing bodies and developing brains. The reality today, however, is that many children have much *worse* nutrition than the adults living in the same home when they actually need *more* nutrition to grow.

Nutrient-deficient children today are setting the stage for a whole new generation of people with chronic disease tomorrow. We cannot ignore that children aren't growing properly. More and more children are taking growth hormone to achieve proper height simply due to the lack of nutrients in their food. They literally are not getting enough to grow. Many of the children I treat grow several inches between visits after merely starting on the correct nutrients. So many children today also have volatile moods and white spots on their nails, which are two obvious signs of nutrient deficiencies.

Vitamin D is a critical nutrient, actually a fat-soluble hormone, that's obtained through exposure to sunlight and diet. The problem with vitamin

D levels today is that more and more people are becoming deficient. The main reason is an increased use of sunblock, which prevents the skin from absorbing vitamin D from sunlight. Even moisturizers today have sunblock, so it's not uncommon for many men and women to effectively never have exposed skin without sunblock, which completely obstructs their ability to make active vitamin D. Ideally, rather than supplementing, I recommend that patients get what Mother Nature intended, which is sunlight without sunblock every day for at least fifteen to twenty minutes per day. After this period of time, you should apply a zinc oxide or titanium dioxide sunscreen to protect your skin from the sun's damaging ultraviolet A (UVA) and ultraviolet B (UVB) rays.

• **Sugar Overload** One reason we're so chronically nutrient deficient is that as a nation, we're eating too much sugar, which takes up the necessary space in our bodies that key nutrients need. Experts estimate that in the 1800s, the average American consumed no more than two pounds of sugar per *year*. Today, the average American consumes nearly 160 pounds of sugar per year. This is almost half a pound a *day*, or nearly forty times higher. Clearly, this is an addiction that needs to stop in order for us to get healthier.[65]

So where does all this sugar come from?

Much of it is hidden in processed foods such as soft drinks, packaged snacks, sweets and desserts, reconstituted meat products like chicken or fish nuggets, and instant noodles and soups.[66] These products make up 58 percent of the calories Americans consume and contribute a whopping 90 percent of the added sugars! Think about this. Most Americans don't even realize that these types of "non-sweet" foods are filled with sugar because they don't taste sweet.

But sugar, no matter where it comes from, is a stressor on the body and causes a dramatic spike in blood sugar, which typically triggers an inflammatory response. Eat it regularly and you're keeping your body in a state of chronic inflammation.

What's more, sugar depresses the immune system for up to six hours after eating it, which means the immune system can't properly do its job after you eat sugar. Imagine now that our diet, which is chock-full of sugar, is keeping our immune system chronically depressed and unable to do its job for long periods of time. And since the immune system is in constant communication with our gut and our vagus nerve, this means a sugar-rich diet is contributing to stress levels and to an imbalance in our microbiome. When you see how everything in the body is interconnected, you begin to understand why so many people today are chronically unwell.

THE PEANUT BUTTER AND JELLY SANDWICH
FIFTY YEARS AGO VS. TODAY

To get a sense of how our food supply has changed, let's look at the basic peanut butter and jelly sandwich and how it's evolved over the years.

Fifty Years Ago The sandwich was made with wheat bread (probably even homemade), homemade or raw peanut butter with zero sugar, where the oil always separated to the top, and grape jelly that was made from real grapes and simple white sugar.

Today The average peanut butter and jelly sandwich is made on either processed white bread with little fiber and plenty of bromide added for extra fluffiness or on wheat bread with more gluten than the body can handle. Next up is processed peanut butter with ample sugar and vegetable oils added (to stop the natural separation of oil), not to mention a heaping serving of salt. Lastly, the grape jelly has little to no real grapes in it but rather high-fructose corn syrup and purple dye.

This one comparison alone sheds light on the food problem in today's modern culture. And there are plenty of other foods where this comparison can be made, such as syrup, cereal, macaroni and cheese, cookies, crackers, and so much more.

TOO MANY STRESSORS: TIPPING OUR SEESAW

The stressors on our bodies are around us all the time. They're in the air we breathe, the water we drink, the food we eat, and the products we use at home, to name the most obvious sources.

The Stressors in Our Food Today

Visualize your body as the most sophisticated car you can buy, needing premium gasoline. For my patients who are children, I use this analogy all the time. Most understand that if we take the car to the gas station and fill it with the wrong type of gas or oil, it won't work optimally and may even break down. The same applies to our bodies. Why would we think we could function at our best when we feed our bodies junk day after day? Yet that's exactly what so many of us do. The result is that at best, we don't feel great but still manage to get through our days. At worst, we become ill with all sorts of conditions and diseases. If we want our bodies to be healthy and strong, we must treat them well. When we don't, they won't run efficiently, if at all. It all starts with our food supply, which is filled with unhealthy additives, preservatives, and chemicals, namely:

• **Chemical sweeteners** like high-fructose corn syrup (also called "fructose" on food labels), aspartame, and those little pink, yellow, and blue packets you see at the center of restaurant tables are all sweeteners created in a lab to be sweeter than what you'd find in nature, without the calories or sugar. But some research has shown that artificial sweeteners confuse the brain, weakening its natural ability to tell you when to stop eating, thereby triggering you to eat more and causing you to gain weight.[67]

Let's take a look at aspartame. It is a well-documented neurotoxin, meaning it is a toxin to the brain and yet it is one of the most pervasive sweeteners in our food supply today. First, it's *two hundred* times sweeter than sugar. If our taste buds become used to a level of sweetness that is two hundred times sweeter than natural sugar, might this create more and more cravings for processed and artificial sugar since natural foods like fruit no longer taste that sweet? What's worse, aspartame is found in everything from diet drinks to sugar-free snacks. It's also omnipresent in almost every single pack of gum and mints available for purchase at checkout counters these days. (Next time you reach for a pack of gum or you buy a pack for your child, take a look at the ingredients label. You're sure to find aspartame on it.)

To understand this detrimental sweetener further, let's look at what aspartame is made of. Its three components, amino acids, aspartic acid, and phenylalanine, create a substance called an excitotoxin because it can overstimulate or excite cells in the body, triggering everything from headaches to cancer. One long-term study conducted at Harvard found a slightly higher cancer risk in men who ingested aspartame.[68] More studies need to be done, but neither children nor adults should be ingesting this additive, even in small amounts. This was the same sweetener that contributed to my own health crisis so many years ago before I knew just how detrimental it was to the body and overall health.

• **Artificial flavors and colorings/dyes** are ubiquitous in processed foods these days, contributing to the unhealthy "stressor" load on the body. One of the most harmful flavor enhancers is MSG, or monosodium glutamate, which is found in many canned vegetables and soups, some processed meats like breakfast sausages, some seasoning packets and salad dressings, and plenty of Chinese food. Like aspartame, MSG has been labeled an excitotoxin, triggering symptoms like headaches, poor attention span, muscle tightness, fatigue, and numbness and/or tingling in the body, as well as irritable bowel syndrome and fibromyalgia. (On labels, it goes by a multitude of names, a few of which are monopotassium glutamate, glutamic acid, calcium cascinate, soy protein and/or soy protein isolate, ajinomoto, and vegetable protein extract.[69])

Anything labeled as "artificial color added" (e.g., red, green, blue, or yellow dye followed by a number) includes food dyes, which are chemicals created in a factory and are pervasive in candy, colored drinks, snacks, and more. And those small bottles of food coloring you add to cookies, cakes, and/or frostings for your child's bake sale? Those are all chemical dyes (unless they specifically say they're nature-based or derived from natural food coloring). Chemical dyes have been linked to hyperactivity and allergic reactions, particularly in kids. On food labels, look for and steer clear of red #40, yellow #5, and yellow #6, which make up about 90 percent of all food dyes.[70]

 Chemical dyes have been linked to hyperactivity and allergic reactions, particularly in kids. On food labels, look for and steer clear of red #40, yellow #5, and yellow #6, which make up about 90 percent of all food dyes.

• **Unhealthy fats** like artificial trans fats (listed as "hydrogenated," "partially hydrogenated," or "fractionated" oils/fats on a food label) and oxidized fats have been exposed to enough heat to cause molecular changes that can cause cellular damage in the body. Avoiding unhealthy fats like canola or rapeseed, cottonseed, corn, and soy oils is a good first step. These fats are abundant in processed foods like cookies and crackers, baked goods like store-bought muffins, donuts, and cakes, stick margarines, and deep-fried foods. Unhealthy fats have absolutely no nutritive value for the body and instead raise bad cholesterol levels (LDL) and lower good cholesterol levels (HDL), which are essential for a healthy heart. This is why, over time, eating trans fats has been shown to increase inflammation in the body, along with increasing the risk of developing heart disease and stroke. Once you stop eating them, your body has less stress to deal with in its struggle to become healthy.

• **Chemical preservatives** are abundant in processed foods, helping to keep foods shelf stable for long periods of time. Some naturally based preservatives exist as well, but overall, if a food can last for years on a shelf without spoiling, you have to ask yourself how that can possibly be good for the body.

In Chapter Two, I mentioned potassium bromate, a substitute for iodine that increases volume in bread products so you get fluffier breads and rolls. This is another chemical preservative you want to avoid. Potassium bromate has been shown to cause cancer, which is why California requires a warning label on products that contain this ingredient. What's more, the International Agency for Research on Cancer determined that potassium bromate is a probable human carcinogen. And by replacing the iodine in bread products and consuming less iodized salt, we are consuming less iodine today than ever, putting us at risk for thyroid disorders and cystic diseases, like cystic breasts, ovarian cysts, and prostate enlargement.[71]

Other chemical preservatives that create a stress load on the body include sodium benzoate or its additive name, E211. This antibacterial and anti-fungal preservative is often added to acidic foods like soda (as carbonic acid), vinegar (as acetic acid), pickles, salsa and dips, and vinegar-based salad dressings. Then there's sodium nitrite, found in most deli meats and processed meats like hot dogs. When added to foods, sodium nitrate forms nitrosamines, substances that may cause cancer. One study in the journal *Nutrition and Cancer* found that eating processed meats, many of which contain these preservatives, exposes people to more carcinogenic compounds, which may be a trigger of colorectal cancer.[72] No one study is ever definitive, but when studies begin to show links, we must pay attention.

• **Pesticides and herbicides** are being used in increasing excess on agricultural crops around the country. As I've mentioned, one of the most powerful and concerning pesticides is glyphosate (the active ingredient in Roundup herbicides), which the World Health Organization has deemed a probable human carcinogen. While nonorganic wheat, corn, and soy crops are sprayed with glyphosate, as well as nonorganic cotton (affecting nonorganic sheets, clothing, and tampons), it can also spread to other food that hasn't been treated with it directly. Even food labeled as organic is not immune, depending on the crop's proximity to a conventionally sprayed farm. For example, organic honey was found to have residues of glyphosate, as were some organic wines.[73] Even if you're eating clean, unprocessed, organic food, which is what I recommend to all my patients to reduce the toxic load on the body, you may still be taking in residues of this powerful toxin, hence the necessity for detoxifying the body on a regular basis.

Our Toxic Food Supply and Disease Rates

There are plenty of statistics that show chronic disease rates have risen steadily as our food supply has changed, and nowhere is this more evident than with type 2 diabetes. With more than twenty-nine million Americans who have the disease and 1.4 million being diagnosed every year, diabetes has become an epidemic in our country.[74] Type 2 diabetes occurs when people have become resistant to the high levels of circulating insulin in their bodies. Insulin is produced by the pancreas to offset sugar consumption. The more sugar consumed, the more insulin is produced. When insulin has been circulating at high levels for long enough, the body essentially becomes immune to it and no longer absorbs the sugar from the blood as it once did in response to insulin. Glucose then circulates at high levels in the blood without being absorbed into the cells and in turn without being processed by the body. This is why the hallmark of diabetes is high blood sugar.

What's more, eighty-four million Americans aged twenty and older have prediabetes, the condition that predisposes people to full-onset diabetes, putting them at risk of other chronic diseases like heart disease.[75] This is simply not normal.

 Eighty-four million Americans aged twenty and older have prediabetes, the condition that predisposes people to full-onset diabetes, putting them at risk of other chronic diseases like heart disease. This is simply not normal.

The bad news is that the number one cause of diabetes is the processed foods we're eating. The good news is that we control what foods we're putting into our bodies, hence we control whether we get diabetes or not. The problem, however, is that we have become accustomed to eating processed and artificial foods as our main food source. Not only does this way of eating contribute to the onset of diabetes, but these foods are some of the top stressors on the body. They are chock-full of ingredients created in factories, ones that we, and our bodies, are not able to recognize (and many of which we aren't even able to pronounce), triggering chronic inflammation. A simple rule to follow: If you can't pronounce the ingredient on the label, then it doesn't belong inside your body. If we all followed this, we could all be significantly healthier.

Not only is what we're eating processed and unhealthy, it's also laden with chemicals, which are toxins. The toxic ingredients in our food supply bombard the body, creating substances that are hard to digest, putting a tremendous burden on the liver and the microbiome and causing potential cell damage over the long term. To give you a sense of how much of these chemicals are in our bodies, research has found 267 toxins in placental blood from pregnant mothers.[76] (The placenta is the barrier for toxic elements being shared between a mother and her baby.) These chemicals are hormonal disruptors that can affect growth and development in babies and children and the normal growth and development of cells in our DNA in adults.

Here's the problem with the chemicals in use today: It's estimated that about eighty-five thousand new chemicals have been created and are in circulation, not only in food but also in personal care products, our home environment, and the environment around us. And only a small percentage of them have been tested for their effects on human health.[77] Under federal law, companies do not have to disclose chemicals or gain approval from the FDA for the products they put on the market every year. The chemicals, if you can believe it, are assumed "safe until proven dangerous." This means the onus of proof is on the sick consumer to prove the chemicals are unhealthy for you, rather than on the company to prove they're good for you before they put them into a product.

FAST FACT It's estimated that about eighty-five thousand new chemicals have been created and are in circulation, not only in food but also in personal care products, our home environment, and the environment around us. And only a small percentage of them have been tested for their effects on human health.

It is therefore up to you to be aware of the ingredients in the food you're eating and in the products you're using, and to be cautious of any ingredients you're not sure of, safety-wise.

Food Sensitivities as Stressors

Unlike a food allergy, which triggers the immune system to immediately attack certain proteins in food as if they were harmful bacteria, viruses, or parasites, often with life-threatening results, a food sensitivity is less immediate and therefore less obvious. But this doesn't mean that it's less harmful to the body.

When someone with a food sensitivity eats an offending food, the immune system is aggravated by that food, triggering inflammation. But rather than mounting an all-out attack, the results are more subtle and long term. Fatigue, headaches, brain fog, persistent dark circles under the eyes (often called "allergic shiners" because they signal an underlying allergy), persistent acne, unexplained skin rashes, gas, and bloating are all typical symptoms I see in patients who are experiencing food sensitivities. These are also referred to as a food intolerance or a non-IGE-mediated food hypersensitivity. These symptoms don't typically occur immediately but instead can happen several hours after eating a food and may persist for several days. If a patient with a food sensitivity eats that food all the time, symptoms are often persistent.

FAST FACT

When someone with a food sensitivity eats an offending food, the immune system is aggravated by that food, triggering inflammation. But rather than mounting an all-out attack, the results are more subtle and long term. Fatigue, headaches, brain fog, persistent dark circles under the eyes (often called "allergic shiners" because they signal an underlying allergy), persistent acne, unexplained skin rashes, gas, and bloating are all typical symptoms I see in patients who are experiencing food sensitivities.

Food intolerances or sensitivities have been steadily increasing over the past thirty years due to our food supply. This should come as no surprise. As food has become more processed and more genetically modified from its original state (e.g., genetically modified corn), with more chemicals being added for flavoring, consistency, and even color, our bodies are unable to recognize the majority of the ingredients and are therefore unable to determine how to process them once they get into our digestive systems. These modern foods may seem to make sense to us (they make our food taste better and/or have fewer calories), but our bodies' digestive systems are biologically primitive. As such, our digestive and immune systems don't learn to interpret these processed ingredients or utilize them. That's why "modern" ingredients like refined starches, sugar, and oxidized and trans fats all trigger chronic inflammation in the body.[78]

One of the key sensitivity culprits today is wheat. The way wheat is grown today is much different than how wheat was grown sixty or even fifty years ago. It's highly processed, contains more of the protein gluten (which adds volume to bread products) than it ever did, and contains fewer minerals than the traditional wheat our grandparents grew up on. Overall, our bodies are unable to recognize the modern wheat that is grown today. A better option is organic heritage wheat, which is made from ancient grains like einkorn, kamut (or Khorasan wheat), and Rouge de Bordeaux. These grains haven't been overprocessed and are not high in gluten. I find that many patients who can't tolerate modern wheat can eat heritage wheat without any problems.

It's no surprise, then, that numbers of people with celiac disease, which is an autoimmune disease where the body's immune system attacks itself when gluten is present, are rising. It's estimated that three million Americans have celiac disease, where the villi (crucial to the absorption of nutrients in the small intestine) are damaged from the body's immune response to gluten.[79] This results in an inability to provide the body and cells with the nutrients they need, which can lead to malnourishment, anemia, dramatic weight loss, and more. In order to truly help patients with celiac, we remove all carbohydrates from their diet for a period of time to let their gut heal.

FAST FACT

It's estimated that three million Americans have celiac disease, where the villi (crucial to the absorption of nutrients in the small intestine) are damaged from the body's immune response to gluten. This results in an inability to provide the body and cells with the nutrients they need, which can lead to malnourishment, anemia, dramatic weight loss, and more.

But for those with celiac, gluten is not the only problem. Once the intestinal wall has been eroded, the patient has lost their ability to digest *all* carbohydrates. Therefore, removing all carbohydrates for a period of time, usually three to six months, restores gut health to ideal levels to ensure optimal absorption of nutrients and microbiome regulation once again. This is the basis of diets like the Specific Carbohydrate Diet (SCD) and Gut and Psychology Syndrome Diet (GAPS). If only gluten is avoided, the patient may no longer have abdominal pain and bloating, but the villi within the gut will not fully heal and therefore neither the microbiome nor digestion will be functioning as well as possible.

Research shows that consumption of modern wheat can increase intestinal permeability even in those who aren't diagnosed with celiac disease.[80] Intestinal permeability is what causes undigested food particles to make their way into the bloodstream, setting off an immune response and subsequent inflammation. This is why one of the first things I tell patients who are obviously suffering from inflammation is to eliminate gluten entirely to aid the healing response of the body and then to slowly reintroduce organic heritage wheat (which is naturally lower in gluten) to see if they can tolerate it. This helps calm the immune system down so I can clearly assess what else is going on in the body. For some, in the end, it is clear that a sensitivity to modern wheat and gluten is what started the whole ball rolling.

I recently treated a young boy named Eric who had spent over a year sick and unable to attend school regularly. He was always complaining of stomach pain, headaches, and fatigue. When he began treatment, I asked him to avoid gluten while I addressed some of the viral and bacterial infections I identified in his blood work. About six months later, he returned with stomachaches, headaches, and fatigue once again, causing him to miss two weeks of school in a row. The difference was that he was back to eating gluten. I explained to Eric and his parents that if Eric completely avoided gluten, he would once again be well. He did, and within the next few weeks he began to improve and returned to school.

Another key sensitivity culprit is dairy, which in countless people triggers inflammation in the gut. For people who don't produce the enzyme lac**tase**, which is required to digest the sugar in dairy called lac**tose**, eating diary is guaranteed to cause digestive upset and inflammation in the body. For others who produce lactase but still experience reactions to milk, yogurt, cheese, and ice cream, their immune systems are most likely reacting to the two proteins in dairy: casein and/or whey. It's estimated that 10 to 20 percent of those who are intolerant to gluten are also intolerant to lactose.[81]

 It's estimated that 10 to 20 percent of those who are intolerant to gluten are also intolerant to lactose.

In addition, most commercially produced non-organic dairy today has hormones and antibiotics added to it, which create more stress on our body and our gut when we consume them. These hormones can trigger hormonal imbalances within the body. For example, as a resident, I had a five-year-old girl producing milk from her nipples after drinking nonorganic milk and eating nonorganic dairy produced with bovine growth hormone (BGH), which is also referred to as recombinant bovine growth hormone (rBGH) or recombinant bovine somatotropin (rBST). BGH is a synthetic hormone injected into dairy cows to make them produce more milk. In humans, it can also stimulate the production of hormones like estrogen, testosterone, and progesterone.[82] I asked the mom to change the girl's milk and dairy to strictly organic and when the girl returned to see me three months later, her lactation had stopped and her breasts had flattened. These kinds of examples have become far too prevalent today, particularly among children, who are experiencing menstruation and puberty much earlier than ever. Again, we need to ask ourselves why this is happening and not allow this to become the new normal.

An unhealthy diet, however, is only one component of food sensitivities. Chronic stress and inflammation in the gut also create abnormal permeability in the intestinal walls, another cause of leaky gut syndrome (read more about this below).[83] The result of leaky gut, no matter what the cause, is that undigested particles of food that shouldn't be in the bloodstream are increasingly leaking into it, setting off an immune storm that includes chronic inflammation, particularly if you continue to eat the offending foods.

Listening to what your body is telling you through symptoms is key when it comes to food sensitivities. If you think you're having a reaction to dairy, wheat, soy, peanuts, or eggs (the five most common food sensitivities), eliminate the suspect food completely from your diet for two weeks and then add it back in slowly. If you experience a response (e.g., gas, bloating, and/or skin rashes), this is your body telling you that you can't tolerate the food and need to eliminate it from your diet. Listening to your body when it comes to food is the first step to optimal health.

LEAKY GUT SYNDROME: HOW IT HAPPENS

Most of the digestion of our food occurs in the small intestine. This is where our gut microbes help digest food and where bile helps break down food, namely fats. The reason is that the small intestine absorbs 90 percent of the nutrients from the food we eat, accomplished by microscopic finger-like projections called villi along the mucus-lined walls.

To give you a sense of the enormity of the villi, consider that every square inch of mucosa in the small intestine, which is about twenty-six feet in length, contains around twenty thousand villi. And, what's more, each one of the cells on the surface of the mucosa of the small intestine contain something called microvilli, which are even smaller finger-like projections. There are about 130 billion microvilli per square inch. All are working together to ensure the proper digestion of food and nutrients and proper filtration of these nutrients (and nothing else) into the body. You may be surprised to learn that about two gallons of food, liquids, and digestive secretions get filtered into our bloodstream for our cells every day.[84] Truly amazing!

In someone with leaky gut syndrome (or intestinal permeability, as it's sometimes called), this process has become flawed because the lining of the small intestine, with all its villi and microvilli working together, has become damaged, allowing undigested food particles, toxins, and bacteria to "leak" into the bloodstream. Researchers have determined that the protein zonulin, which is needed to "seal" gut cells together in the form of tight junctions, is compromised in leaky gut, allowing for the cells to "unseal" and become gap junctions that "leak."[85] Since 70 percent of your immune system is found in the gut, this permeability triggers tremendous inflammation in the gut and in the body, creating symptoms from regular bloating and gas to fatigue, food sensitivities, and even skin rashes.

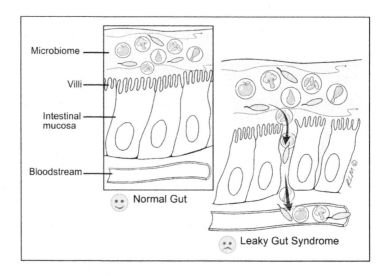

Microbiome

Villi

Intestinal mucosa

Bloodstream

Normal Gut

Leaky Gut Syndrome

Leaky gut has yet to acquire a true clinical "label" today. The closest to leaky gut is irritable bowel syndrome or IBS, but this is diagnosed only when there is pain, bloating, diarrhea, and/or constipation. Most cases of leaky gut don't present with obvious gastrointestinal symptoms, but they do contribute to most other clinical conditions. In fact, one could argue today that most chronic conditions begin with a leaky gut, since it is the dysregulation of the microbiome that sets the stage for illness to result. The gut is where health begins. If there is excessive inflammation in a patient's gut, it translates to compromised immunity. There are also most likely digestion issues, neurological disease, mental illness, behavioral problems, autoimmune disease, and more.

Environmental Toxins as Stressors

The concept of environmental toxins can feel overwhelming, particularly since we have little to no control over so many of them. Airborne toxins are assaulting us in record numbers, and pollution in our water is on the rise. Heavy metals are also found just about everywhere. Let's take a closer look at each of these types of toxins in the following sections and explore what we can do to counteract them.

• **Toxins in the air** account for the majority of environmental pollutants today. Because we no longer see the smog of the industrial era in most cities, we assume our air quality is fine, but sadly, this is not true. Studies have shown that heavy metals, namely aluminum, mercury, arsenic, cadmium, and lead, permeate our air as the result of use in industry, farming, and at home. The pesticides sprayed on lawns and gardens, both in public places and at home, are but one example. One study describes these heavy metals in this way: "These metallic elements are considered systemic toxicants that are known to induce multiple organ damage, even at lower levels of exposure. They are also classified as human carcinogens (known or probable) according to the US Environmental Protection Agency and the International Agency for Research on Cancer."[86]

The majority of us don't want to wear a mask everywhere we go, so how do we avoid these outdoor pollutants? The short answer is that for the most part, we can't. What we can do, however, is cease using toxic chemicals in our own yards and gardens in favor of more nature-based solutions.

Not all airborne toxins, however, are found outdoors. Mold, chemicals, and volatile organic compounds (VOCs) also pervade the indoor environments of our homes and offices. What makes this indoor pollution worse is that our homes and offices are often "sealed" up, which makes our indoor air quality worse.

One of these VOCs is perchloroethylene (also known as tetrachloroethylene, PCE, or PERC). This is the chemical released into the air after you dry-clean your clothes and also remains on your clothes after dry cleaning (it's even been found to concentrate on clothing with repeated dry cleanings). Long-term exposure to PERC has been found to trigger neurological impairment; kidney, liver, and reproductive problems; and cancer, particularly bladder cancer, non-Hodgkin's lymphoma, and multiple myeloma.[87] The problem with PERC is that while it starts as a liquid, it vaporizes or evaporates into the air, which you can't see or feel but you breathe in. Research has found that this evaporation intensifies with heat—say, for instance, after you pick up your dry cleaning and leave it a hot car for hours. Better options for your health include CO_2 cleaning, which uses liquid carbon dioxide not traditional solvents to clean clothes, and wet cleaning, which uses water and biodegradable soaps. Hand-washing clothes is always an option too.

Chemical air fresheners and chemical fragrances also contribute to the problem. Just as with chemical flavors in food, these chemical scents are not natural to our bodies and once inside the nose, the body often doesn't know what to do with them. Not only are potent scents frequently a trigger for headaches or even nausea in highly sensitive people, but when breathed in, the liver has to detoxify the ingredients or they get stored in the extracellular matrix.

Research has shown that fragranced consumer products emit a range of volatile organic compounds that can affect air quality and health. One small study conducted at the University of Washington found that scented laundry detergents and dryer sheets contain more than twenty-five volatile air pollutants, including the carcinogens acetaldehyde and benzene, and release them into the air through the dryer vent. According to the American Cancer Society, benzene causes leukemia and other blood cancers, while acetaldehyde has been linked to nasal and throat cancers. This is why I recommend switching from conventional to naturally derived detergents, fabric softeners, and other home cleaning products. They're simply healthier for us.[88]

I am not suggesting that we become a scentless environment or never use scented products. There simply needs to be a limit. For example, if we use three different fragrances through various products like body wash, body lotion, and hair styling products, and we have scented homes, cars, offices, and even garbage bags, it starts to tip our seesaw a bit. Moderation with fragrance is key, and just as with food, ingredients that are as close to what Mother Nature has provided are better for you. This is why I recommend organic, simple personal care routines that include naturally derived essential oils for scents (both home and personal) or no scent at all.

• **Toxins in our water supply** have been a growing issue for decades. Our drinking water is simply not clean. What follows are the cold, hard facts about the water filtered into the majority of homes in America.

To begin with, scientists have increasingly found numerous chemicals from pharmaceuticals like opioids, antibiotics, antidepressants, chemotherapy drugs, and heart medications present in our water supply. Since our bodies metabolize only a small portion of the drugs we take, the rest is excreted through urine, feces, or sweat. This is how pharmaceuticals make their way into wastewater, which is eventually treated to become our drinking water. But our treatment plants do not get rid of prescription medications in the water, which is why they end up in our bodies and in the bodies of the fish that we eat. Not only does this hold true for medications we ingest but also for those that are applied. Case in point: Research has estimated that one man's use of testosterone cream can put as much testosterone into the water supply as the natural excretions from three hundred men. Do we really want to be exposed to, or have our children exposed to, hormones in our bath or shower? Definitely not. But this is happening.[89]

FAST FACT

Research has estimated that one man's use of testosterone cream can put as much testosterone into the water supply as the natural excretions from three hundred men. Do we really want to be exposed to, or have our children exposed to, hormones in our bath or shower? Definitely not. But this is happening.

Water is sacred, and clean water free of toxins is essential to our health. But our water supply is being contaminated every single day, so our bodies have to attempt to cope. As scientist Masaru Emoto says in *The Hidden Messages of Water* (see page 83), toxins destroy water's natural structure, thereby not quenching our bodies' thirst for what it really needs: clean water from natural, unpolluted springs.[90]

This is clearly illustrated with a four-year-old patient of mine who was refusing to drink water. When I asked the child's mother to tell me exactly what kind of water she was being offered, she told me it was water filtered through reverse osmosis. This filter purifies toxins from water but results in water that's acidic and lacks minerals. Because this young patient has a disease of the joints called juvenile rheumatoid arthritis, which is often characterized by high levels of inflammation and acid in the body, it stands to reason that this little girl didn't want to drink acidic water. I asked her mother to offer mineral water instead, which is alkaline. After she bought the water, her daughter took a taste and started drinking right away. Amazingly, this four-year-old's body instinctively recognized exactly what was best for her. These kinds of situations sound unbelievable because the answers are sometimes so simplistic. But after drinking water again, and after being treated at my clinic for infections and mold exposure, this young girl now no longer has juvenile rheumatoid arthritis.

I realize that not everyone can afford to filter their entire home or drink nothing but mineral water out of glass bottles (which is the optimum scenario), so we must simply do the best we can. I suggest that whenever possible, you drink the purest water you have access to and avoid bottled water in BPA plastic. (BPA is one chemical we know about, but there are plenty more used in packaging, the health effects of which we have yet to discover.) Beyond that, a shower filter and a tap filter are two ways to cut down on exposure.

And what about the polluted waters where we get the fish we eat? While it's nearly impossible to avoid these toxins, we must simply do our best. Certain waters are cleaner than others, but at this point, it's probably safe to assume that we're ingesting some degree of pollutants whenever we eat seafood. This doesn't mean we shouldn't eat fish. It simply means we should eat it in moderation and be mindful of its source. I have found that the Environmental Working Group is a reliable source of healthy living advice, including seafood choices.

• **Heavy metals** such as mercury, aluminum, lead, nickel, tin, cadmium, titanium, arsenic, and antimony are becoming prolific in our soil, our water, our personal care products, and the air we breathe. Why is this problematic? Enzymes, which are critical for the chemical reactions within every cell of the body, work optimally if a mineral such as potassium, selenium, sodium, or magnesium are bound to them. But if there are no minerals, they will find something to bind to instead, even toxic heavy metals like aluminum, lead, mercury, and cadmium. This is why it's important to maintain optimum mineral levels in the body. Not only do minerals keep our enzymes working optimally but they also prevent our enzymes from binding to and locking heavy metals into the body. When this happens, the metal begins to accumulate in our tissues instead of being detoxified by the liver and excreted from the body. As the heavy metal burden increases, our enzymes become more and more disabled.

What's more, different heavy metals prefer different organs of the body. Aluminum, for example, prefers to accumulate in the brain, as researchers have found when studying Alzheimer's disease.[91] Mercury also prefers the brain and is able, as some scientists have found, to actually circumvent the blood-brain barrier meant to keep toxins out of the brain. Other metals like cadmium and lead gravitate to the bone marrow.[92]

FAST FACT

Different heavy metals prefer different organs of the body. Aluminum, for example, prefers to accumulate in the brain, as researchers have found when studying Alzheimer's disease. Mercury also prefers the brain and is able, as some scientists found, to actually circumvent the blood-brain barrier meant to keep toxins out of the brain. Other metals like cadmium and lead gravitate to the bone marrow.

Now, you're probably asking, why has this heavy metal absorption become a bigger health issue today than ever before? The answer is simple. Because our soil is so depleted of the minerals that our body needs to naturally bind to enzymes, we're all more mineral deficient. This means that the enzymes in our bodies are binding more often to heavy metals, rather than much-needed minerals, triggering a greater toxic burden on our bodies. This causes everything from cognitive decline and reduced processing speed to ADHD, osteoporosis, and high blood pressure. Heavy metal burden is pervasive and more problematic for our health than most people realize. In fact, I would argue that almost all chronic diseases today have an element of heavy metal burden that is not being considered in the current management of these diseases.

Personal Care Products as Stressors

We've come a long way from the days of using simple soap (often handmade) and water on our skin. Granted, many of our personal care products today accomplish much more than plain old soap and water ever did. They keep skin (including lips) hydrated for twenty-four hours or more, delay the onset of fine lines and wrinkles, prevent sunburn, get rid of acne, slough off dead skin cells, and so much more. But we have to ask, *At what cost?*

And then there are the toothpastes, makeup, sunscreens, bug repellants, and fragrances we spray or roll on, often using these products more than once a day. When we combine these with our skincare products, the result is a toxic overload on the body.

Numerous personal care products today are manufactured to be more "effective" and, in the case of skincare products, specifically designed to better penetrate the skin's barrier with so-called "nanotechnology." However, many of these substances—some of which, like chemical-based sunscreens and bug repellants, contain toxic chemicals—are designed to get into and past the skin's barrier function, bypassing the body's first line of immune defense. This is how these ingredients make their way into the body and more specifically, into the blood.

Chemical sunscreens go by names like oxybenzone, octinoxate, homosalate, octisalate, and octocrylene. These can make their way into the bloodstream and have been shown to disrupt hormones in the body.[93] Better sunscreen bets include physical sunblocks that are free of harmful chemicals. These contain non-nano zinc oxide and titanium dioxide.

We must also keep in mind that some makeup, including kohl eyeliners and eyeshadows, as well as lipsticks and lip glosses, have been shown to contain lead, the toxic mineral I discussed earlier. Other makeup has been shown to potentially contain the cancer-causing chemical asbestos. The amounts of lead have sometimes been enough to trigger lead poisoning in small children. (This is why I always recommend to parents that they read and recognize the ingredients in makeup that they and their children use, including Halloween makeup.) In the case of lip products, it was found that many contain trace amounts of lead (about 1 mg/kg, a unit used to measure concentrations of chemicals). To be clear, the Food and Drug Administration states that this amount of lead in lipstick is not enough to "pose a health risk." But if you're one to apply and reapply lipstick (or lip balm, including ones with SPF) all day long, you want to be sure yours is as toxin-free as possible. (The reason you have to continue to reapply lipstick is that you're inadvertently ingesting some of it.)[94]

113

Chemical preservatives called parabens, phthalates (chemicals that can disrupt the body's hormonal system), synthetic colors and fragrances, triclosan (an antimicrobial chemical), and formaldehyde (an antibacterial chemical) are all ingredients that could potentially irritate sensitive skin, not to mention the body. And once these ingredients get into the body, the body has to detox them through the liver.

 Chemical preservatives called parabens, phthalates (chemicals that can disrupt the body's hormonal system), synthetic colors and fragrances, triclosan (an antimicrobial chemical), and formaldehyde (an antibacterial chemical) are all ingredients that could potentially irritate sensitive skin, not to mention the body.

This is not to say you should never wear makeup or fragrance or use skin-care products to delay the effects of aging. What is critical, as with food, is to read the labels, know the ingredients in the products you're using, and use personal care products in moderation.

As with everything, keeping the body in an optimal state of balance is critical to overall health. If you're not eating a well-balanced diet, not living a healthy lifestyle, and have a microbiome that's severely out of balance, it's not a great idea to add to your body's already challenged load. You'll only contribute to your body and your seesaw becoming even more out of balance. But, if you're generally healthy, then using some of these products should be fine, in moderation. As I mentioned earlier, however, knowing and understanding the ingredients you're putting onto and into your body is a critical step you can take toward optimal health.

Invisible Toxins: Radio Frequency Energy as a Stressor

Radio frequency (RF) energy is a form of electromagnetic energy that's part of the electromagnetic spectrum. This includes microwaves, visible light, and X-rays, as well as RF emissions, waves, and/or fields, which occur when a transmitter is fed to an antenna. Radio frequency energy represents

WHY YOU SHOULD AVOID HAND SANITIZERS

Everyone, it seems, has hand sanitizer stashed in their bags, their cars, their homes, and their offices to get rid of germs and bacteria before they can make us sick. But the truth is that our obsession with hand sanitizers is making us even sicker by giving rise to stronger, more resistant bugs and bacteria. This is thanks to antibiotic ingredients in hand sanitizers like triclosan and triclocarban, which kill good bacteria along with the bad, making you more susceptible to illness in the long run.

Triclosan, also found in some toothpastes, deodorants, hair products, and cosmetics, has also been found to disrupt hormones in the body.[123] For these reasons, I always advise my patients to avoid hand sanitizers and antibacterial soaps and wash their hands with good old soap and warm water. What's more, some bacteria and germs are actually good for you, as long as you're not immunocompromised. These bugs can stimulate your immune system to become even stronger.

a bimodal sign wave, meaning a wave form that has an up-down pattern in two dimensions only, unlike natural waves from the sun and earth, which have three dimensions.

Cell phones, for example, use radio frequency energy. While there has been a debate on the effect of this energy on the body, we do know from recent scientific observations that it's becoming more of a stressor. Some studies have actually proven the negative effects of radio frequency on the body, namely that this type of energy can affect cell behavior, particularly within the nervous system.[95] There are skeptics, of course, who question this, but as I've emphasized throughout the book, each individual person and their seesaw is different. While RF energy may not affect some people's seesaws, it can be incredibly difficult for others to cope with, particularly those with neurological disease.

Some studies have actually proven the negative effects of radio frequency on the body, namely that this type of energy can affect cell behavior, particularly within the nervous system.

This is why I encourage *all* patients to reduce, if not completely remove, exposure to radio frequency energy while sleeping. The nervous system is a highly tuned circuit breaker and is completely dependent on frequency and electrical signals. Therefore, when it rests, it needs to truly rest (i.e., not be bombarded by extra frequency all night long that keeps it on high alert). In order for the body to heal, it needs to rejuvenate. For the nervous system, this means powering down completely. When patients are able, I recommend that they unplug their wireless router just before bed. Turning off cell phones and computers before bed helps too.

THE GROWING TOXIC BURDEN ON THE BODY

The stressors that are causing our bodies to tip out of balance are quite different from what was stressing our bodies fifty years ago. Modern stressors include chronic and acute infections, the overaccumulation of biofilms and dysregulation of our microbiome, liver stress from too many toxins, pharmaceutical drug metabolism, unhealthy diets, poor water quality, and radiation exposure in the form of electromagnetic fields (EMFs). Yet nowhere in the medical paradigm today are these things being considered. Why is that?

There are hundreds of current research articles that describe the growing burden of toxicity on our bodies as the "chemical body burden."[96] These are the number of chemicals that, rather than being metabolized or excreted, are stored in human tissue. Yet there is no active treatment of toxins within medicine today. I see this every day in my medical practice: chronically sick patients whose bodies are tipped too far in one direction because of the incredible toxin load they're dealing with. What makes it challenging is that even if every patient were to be exposed to the same toxic chemicals, they would exhibit different symptoms or at varied intervals because every body is unique. In other words, these epigenetic effects are expressed differently in different patients, making individualization of care important.

A DAY IN THE LIFE OF MODERN-DAY STRESSORS

NIGHTIME Overnight, we release growth hormones while we're sleeping, which, when we get restorative sleep, activates tissue regeneration. In fact, the production of melatonin (the hormone that regulates sleep and is essential for the release of growth hormones) by the pineal gland is dependent on complete darkness. Those of us who have "blue lights" (electronics like computers and cell phones emit blue light, as do fluorescent and LED bulbs) in the bedroom are at risk for not secreting optimal levels of melatonin because these lights tell the pineal gland it is still light out and in turn, suppress the secretion of melatonin. This is where some health problems may begin.

All night long, we're also breathing in the air of our homes. If our homes have mold that produces mycotoxins (toxic chemicals produced by fungi) or volatile organic compounds (VOCs, chemical gases given off by a wide variety of products), what happens then?

Fifty years ago, homes were ventilated largely with fresh air through windows and fans. Basement and attic air remained in those areas and didn't travel to other parts of the house. I still remember my grandmother opening the windows every day as part of her morning ritual, both winter and summer. Today, however, the majority of homes have forced air and the windows remain closed. This means that whatever is in our basements or attics is being "forced" through our homes for us to breathe all the time. Most of us are in the dark about the air quality in our basements or attics, or worse, we know there are issues with water damage, but because they are "out of sight, out of mind," we don't realize we're breathing in this air.

Instead of regenerating, our bodies have had to detoxify all night.

MORNING Hopefully, when we wake, we start the day with a large glass of *clean* water, but unfortunately, the municipal water supply today has more and more detrimental toxins in it, from pharmaceutical residue to manufacturing runoff to heavy metals. All of these are represented in "safe" levels, but even so, why would we want to drink it? The best water put into our bodies should be completely clean. Yet we either drink tap water, which is sterile but not clean, or we drink a large cup of coffee to get us going. This immediately makes our tissues acidic, which then makes it harder for our bodies to detoxify.

Perhaps worse, those who don't eat breakfast (which is, incredibly, thirty-one million Americans[97]) begin their day's work on an empty stomach. For others, they ingest a quick toaster pastry or muffin filled with gluten and sugar. How is the body supposed to stay strong and power through a healthy day with this kind of start?

MIDDAY Some move into their lunchtimes by eating processed food, too much gluten, which causes more inflammation in our gut, and soda, which is laden with sugar and high-fructose corn syrup or, in the case of diet soda, chemical sweeteners like aspartame.

It's not uncommon for a patient to tell me that they are exhausted by 4:00 p.m. With little to no nourishment and nothing but toxins to process, it becomes very hard to stay energetic and well.

EVENING Time-crunched Americans eat dinner on the go. For others, it's takeout or quick-heat frozen foods. Very few cook healthy meals at home, which include a clean source of protein (e.g., soaked legumes, a variety of grass-fed and/or free-range meats, and/or wild fish with low mercury), a vegetable or two, and a whole-grain or seed-based carbohydrate such as quinoa, millet, or wild rice.

After that meal, it's back to bed again, frequently with sleeplessness, for another night of the body struggling to detox. It's interesting to note that if you awaken every night at a certain time, the reason why may be answered by Traditional Chinese Medicine (TCM). According to what's called the Chinese meridian chart, the body has a natural biological rhythm that it follows, with each organ having its own corresponding time frame. Regularly waking up at a certain time, according to this chart, helps point to where the body is struggling:

Gallbladder time 11:00 p.m.–1:00 a.m.

Liver time 1:00 a.m.–3:00 a.m.

Lung time 3:00 a.m.–5:00 a.m.

Large intestine time 5:00 a.m.–7:00 a.m.

Stomach time 7:00 a.m.–9:00 a.m.

With a typical daily routine that includes many of these unhealthy habits, and without the proper balancers to rebalance our seesaws, it's no wonder our bodies are struggling.

SAME STRESSOR = DIFFERENT SYMPTOMS

The details of why a patient is presenting with certain symptoms lies in their own unique story: their seesaw, what toxins they've been exposed to, and how their health has unfolded. Let's take, for example, a headache. If a headache is managed with a label—a migraine, a tension headache, a chronic daily headache—then the individual circumstances that triggered the headache in a particular patient are being completely disregarded. The headache is only viewed in terms of the type of medication(s) that will quiet the symptoms. But patients get headaches for all different reasons. For some people, headaches are the result of dehydration. They're simply not drinking enough water. For some, it can be cervical subluxation; seeing a chiropractor or a deep tissue massage therapist can help release this tension. For some, it is an indicator of gluten intolerance or other yet undetected food sensitivity. For some, it

119

represents an undiscovered infection in the body. If these reasons aren't explored, giving medication is like trying to disable the smoke detector to stop it from sounding the alarm.

Another growing example of this phenomena is GERD, or gastroesophageal reflux disease, cases of which are on the rise. It's estimated that 20 percent of the population in the United States reports acid reflux symptoms that occur weekly, a number that has doubled in the past decade. Why is this? Our intestinal tracts are under siege today from a glut of food additives, pesticide and herbicide exposure, antibiotics and other medications, low mineral states in the body, and the list goes on. It's no wonder that more people are experiencing reflux, even infants and children. (The number of infants with GERD symptoms who were hospitalized increased by 42 percent, and the number of children between the ages of two and seventeen who were hospitalized for GERD symptoms has increased 84 percent.)[98]

FAST FACT The number of infants with GERD symptoms who were hospitalized increased by 42 percent, and the number of children between the ages of two and seventeen who were hospitalized for GERD symptoms has increased 84 percent.

One of the clearest indicators that something is grossly wrong with the microbiome's development today is when infants develop reflux. From the beginning of time, reflux in infants has been rare. Colic has been common, but not reflux. But the staggering rise in infant reflux is a very loud smoke detector, trying to alert us that we are doing something significantly wrong with our health and how we manage it.

Many patients with GERD have been told it is due to a faulty sphincter muscle and that the symptoms are inevitable. For a very small number with a hiatal hernia, this may in fact be true. But for most, GERD is simply the consequence of food choices, a dysregulated microbiome, and a poorly optimized enterohepatic circulation, meaning digestive juices aren't flowing properly and can be successfully corrected without medication.

If this condition is to be truly corrected, a modern view of how the gastrointestinal or GI tract works and flows is needed, along with a global view of which stressors on the body are triggering this condition. Reflux is caused when food remains in the stomach longer than usual and putrefies. Since this is not normal, we should be looking at *why* this is happening, *why* the normal digestive process isn't working, rather than giving medication to treat the symptoms. All doctors can logically understand this, but we are simply not trained in medical school to think this way in how we approach patients. What's encouraging, though, is that we *all* can approach symptoms, disease, and health in a new way.

CHRONIC INFLAMMATION ON THE RISE

The growing toxic burden on the body is contributing to the high rates of inflammation today, which is in turn depressing our immune system. Some inflammation is healthy, but chronic 24/7 inflammation is not. And that's where we are today as a nation. Chronic inflammation triggers a chronic state of unwell by stressing and injuring cells, causing them to malfunction and age long before their time. This is turn contributes to chronic disease and is significantly reducing our quality of life. There are many causes of chronic inflammation today.

• **Weight gain triggers inflammation in the body.** We sadly are a nation of overweight and obese people and the numbers are on the rise. But people don't realize that fat *causes* inflammation. It is both the *product* of inflammation and also a source.

It's actually pretty simple: lose weight and inflammation decreases. One study at the Fred Hutchinson Cancer Research Center in Seattle, Washington, found that when overweight or obese women dropped pounds (at least 5 percent or more of their body weight), they had measurable declines in markers of inflammation.[99] Weight around the middle, in particular, is an active source of hormones and inflammatory compounds, making it much worse than fat that's evenly distributed.

Exercising moderately also reduces inflammation and keeps your weight down. In addition, a University of Illinois study found that exercise seems to help heal chronic inflammation in the skin, a benefit that could be extrapolated to the entire body, say the researchers. The study, published in the *American Journal of Physiology*, found that exercise helps increase blood flow and decreases the number of inflammatory molecules released in the body. Another study found that just 2.5 hours of moderate exercise per week (about twenty minutes a day) reduced markers of inflammation by 12 percent.[100] This is likely due to the detoxifying effects of sweat. Sweat is considered a "third kidney" and greatly enhances our ability to remove heavy metals, mold toxins, and other water-soluble toxins from our bodies.

• **Food sensitivities are at an all-time high.** As we've discussed, when the gut isn't digesting food properly, undigested food particles leak through the intestinal walls and into the bloodstream. The immune system wages an all-out war to attack the undigested food particles, which it sees as invaders. With this response comes inflammation. The problem is that these food sensitivities are not being diagnosed, so people continue to eat the offending foods without realizing they're the cause of their symptoms (frequent headaches, skin rashes, gas, insomnia, etc.), so the inflammation continues nonstop.

By aiding patients in listening to their bodies, I've been able to help them determine the offending foods and adjust their diets accordingly. The symptoms go away and the inflammation recedes.

• **Chronic stress is overloading the body.** Some stress is okay, but chronic stress keeps levels of stress hormones high in the body, which triggers a state of chronic inflammation. The irony is that even though our overall standard of living today may be higher than in the past, we're more stressed than ever before. As part of our healing process, we must begin to ask ourselves the hard questions about what is stressing us and how we can make changes in order to reduce stress and begin healing.

One other aspect of stress is lack of proper breathing. As mentioned earlier, deep, diaphragmatic breathing is critical to calming the nervous system and the brain, as well as helping to balance our microbiome. Healing starts with taking proper deep belly breaths, not shallow chest breaths. (To learn the proper relaxation breath, see page 162.)

• **Sleep problems are putting the body on high alert.** Insomnia and sleeplessness are on the rise as people are working more and taking less time for themselves. Scientists at Emory University School of Medicine in Atlanta, Georgia, found that sleep deprivation or poor sleep quality raises inflammation in the body.[101] Getting enough sleep not only recharges the body, it also decreases inflammatory hormones like cortisol and adrenaline, which are stress hormones that make the body more susceptible to inflammation.

• **Chronic infections are on the rise.** Research shows that dental infections trigger chronic inflammation in the body that has been linked to diseases like breast cancer and coronary artery disease.[102] These dental infections often occur from root canals not performed properly with the foci of the infection remaining at the root of the tooth, which the patient can no longer feel since the root has been removed. This allows for a slow, chronic leak of infection into the bloodstream, triggering chronic inflammation. This type of inflammation has been directly linked to heart health, since the veins of the mouth drain directly into heart circulation. This is how and why dental infections have been shown to be linked to coronary artery disease.

You may also be surprised to learn that the mouth has its own microbiome, complete with biofilms. Everything that negatively affects the gut microbiome also negatively affects the oral microbiome. The larger consideration, however, is how our oral health affects our total body health.

Allowing bad bacteria, which forms itself into plaque, to proliferate can result in dental bacteria spreading throughout the body. This is why dental and gum care are a critical part of optimal health. You cannot be healthy with a mouth full of rotting teeth and/or gums.

If we are to return our bodies to a state of optimal wellness, we must look at the sources of inflammation in our lives and do our best to mitigate them so they don't tip our seesaws out of balance.

PART IV

A Nation of Well

The natural healing force within each one of us is the greatest force in getting well.

—Hippocrates

5

Balancing the Seesaw: What Keeps Us Well

As I've discussed throughout this book, each one of us has to achieve a state of balance in our bodies every day for optimal health, which is in fact what our bodies are designed to achieve given the right conditions. Anything less and our bodies begin to develop symptoms of imbalance, calling out for help.

Imagine for a moment seeing someone in distress, asking for help. Your first instinct would be to reach out a hand, to do anything to help that person, right? Now imagine symptoms are your body's first calls for help: your gut bacteria are out of balance, your microbiome is shifting, your liver is inflamed, your immune system is laboring. There are easy ways to reach out and get your struggling body back into balance. It's not merely a myth that optimal health can be achieved for each and every one of us. This is my experience *every day*, seeing success in the thousands of patients I have treated over the ten-plus years I've been in practice.

The achievement of optimal health, however, commands a new way of medical thought and practice. It takes listening to and understanding what the body requires in order to be in balance and then giving it what it needs. This is the simple seesaw concept I've been talking about and is one that we must embrace to stem the upward trend of chronic diseases spiraling out of control and threatening to overwhelm our current healthcare system.

Making sure your body has the necessary balancers is a key aspect to staying healthy. These balancers allow the cells and organs in your body to function with peak efficiency, so it's better able to handle whatever toxins and other challenges come its way. The good news is that the body has a phenomenal ability to spontaneously detoxify and rebalance. In fact, some people are able to naturally recover from what ails them, which is why their headaches go away or their rash clears up or they begin to sleep through the night again. Many times, however, the body is unable to do this because it doesn't have the proper nutrients and other balancers to do so.

The bottom line here is that in order to maintain wellness, each of us must get the nutrients we require to keep our cells healthy. It's not nearly as difficult as you may think. Eating a healthy daily diet provides the body with many of the essential vitamins, minerals, and other nutrients (like protein and healthy fats) that it needs to keep its seesaw balanced. The caveat is that once this seesaw has been thrown out of whack, it's harder to supplement with food alone. At this point, the body's deficiencies are often greater than what a daily diet can provide and this, as I have found with so many of my patients, is when supplementation becomes necessary. However, I always recommend people discuss what they need with their doctor and/or a registered dietitian first to make sure they're getting what they need. Too much of a supplement is sometimes just as bad as not getting enough of it.

With this said, the following recommendations (and those in "Your Two-Week Health-Boosting Plan," page 155) are necessary for the body's natural balancers—the gut, the microbiome, the liver, and the immune system—to work with peak efficiency.

1. EAT FARM TO TABLE

My advice is always to eat closer to nature, and straight from the garden (i.e., farm to table) is always best. There's plenty of research to show that people who eat a diet rich in fruits and vegetables have less risk of chronic disease, such as cardiovascular disease and cancer. In fact, researchers have found that there is a "statistically significant protective effect of fruit and vegetable consumption" against cancer.[103] When you think about it, it makes perfect sense. This is what nature provides for us.

If you can't eat farm to table all the time, and I understand that despite the best intentions, many of us can't realistically achieve this in our busy lives, then make it a point to always buy products with six ingredients or fewer, all of which you should be able to recognize and pronounce. These foods should have none of the harmful additives (such as high-fructose corn syrup, aspartame, and chemical food dyes) we've discussed throughout this book. This is what works for my patients and my family, and it will work for you too. In fact, when it comes to food and my own children, I have two simple rules. When they ask whether they can have something or not, I respond by asking if they can (1) pronounce everything on the label and know what it is, and (2) find those ingredients in our home pantry. If the answer is yes to both, they can have the food. If not, they can't. There's no compromise because I know that our food choices affect the entire balance of our seesaw and our health. I ask all my patients, even my youngest ones and their parents, to follow these rules. Guiding our children to learn what foods can help nourish their bodies is something that will help them and their health for a lifetime.

How to eat closer to nature Select organic whenever possible. Part of eating farm to table is eating organic foods, which are closer to the foods our grandparents and their parents ate when chronic diseases were less rampant. Organic foods are lower in pesticide residues and preservatives and are higher in important nutrients and natural chemicals called phytonutrients.

When fruits and vegetables are produced organically without pesticides, these plants actually produce more of these phytonutrients in an effort to help retard insects, fungi, germs, bugs, and other threats to their survival. In fact, organic foods are highest in these phytonutrients (namely carotenoids and flavonoids) *because* of their need for self-defense. They're also higher in the key nutrients vitamin C, iron, magnesium, and phosphorus.[104] It's these nutrients, along with the powerful phytonutrients described below, that help keep the body's seesaw in balance, allowing us to avoid disease.

Carotenoids give red, yellow, and orange colors to fruits like mangos, oranges, cantaloupes, and apricots and to vegetables like carrots, sweet potatoes, bell peppers, and butternut squash. (The deeper the hue, the higher the concentration of phytonutrients, something that holds true for most of these natural chemicals.) One of the key carotenoids is lycopene, which imparts the red or pink hue to watermelon, tomatoes, papaya, guava, and red grapefruit. This particular phytonutrient has been shown to have numerous health benefits, particularly helping to prevent cancer.[105] Other key carotenoids, lutein and zeaxanthin, are found in spinach, kale, and arugula and are important for eye health. (Lutein and zeaxanthin are naturally occurring pigments found in the human eye, but they must be acquired from our diet.)

Flavonoids are phytonutrients that go by names like quercetin (found in produce such as onions, apples, and grapes) and catechins (found in green tea, red wine, and dark chocolate). The health benefits of flavonoids are numerous, namely that they've been found to have anti-inflammatory and anticarcinogenic properties.[106] Anthocyanins are one type of flavonoid that give blue and purple fruits, such as blueberries, blackberries, eggplant, plums, and purple grapes, their rich hue. There are plenty of health reasons to add anthocyanins to your diet. These phytonutrients have been shown to have powerful anti-inflammatory and antimicrobial effects, which may be key to why they help to keep us healthy.[107]

Needless to say, these phytonutrients are not only good for plants, they're good for us as well. Just as phytonutrients help plants protect against threats to their survival, so too do they help ward off potential threats to *our* survival. Bottom line: these are powerful natural chemicals at work and are all the more reason why eating a farm-to-table diet rich in fruits and vegetables will help keep our health seesaw in balance.

Also part of a farm-to-table diet: eating organic, unrefined whole grains. Healthier options include heritage wheat, amaranth, buckwheat, millet, quinoa, rice (brown is preferable, as it has more nutrients like fiber), and wild rice. Oats tend to be high in mycotoxins, which is why I'm cautious about recommending anyone eat them daily. These mycotoxins produced by fungi grow quickly on oat grasses while growing in fields and during storage. All they need are high temperatures and moisture content. Therefore, limiting your intake of oats to once a week and rotating with other whole grains is optimal.

Healthy fats are also essential to keeping your seesaw in balance, as they're necessary for initiating chemical reactions in the body that control growth, immune function, and reproduction—as well as absorbing, storing, and carrying fat-soluble vitamins like A, D, E, and K wherever and whenever cells need them, serving as a source of stored energy. This is how we're able to regulate our energy levels throughout the day. Fats are also critical for brain health and healthy neurotransmission, the lightning-fast communication that occurs between cells in the body. Fats are not only a critical part of brain matter but they also make up myelin, the fatty material that wraps around our nerve cells, helping transmit messages throughout the body. They also regulate body temperature and are necessary for the production of steroid hormones like estrogen and testosterone. These are all reasons why, without a source of healthy fats in our diet, our cells simply cannot function properly. A few healthy fat options are avocados, coconut oil, extra virgin olive oil, ghee (clarified butter devoid of milk proteins), and grass-fed butter, which is higher in healthy omega-3 fatty acids and vitamin K_2 than butter from grain-fed cows.[108]

When it comes to eating healthfully, you don't need a miracle diet to get started. Simply plan to start eating farm to table from this moment forward. Read the food labels and reject any food that you know isn't healthy for your body. Remember that the body and cells are craving real food. Once you start eating organic foods closer to nature, you'll feel the difference (e.g., more energy, sounder sleep, less anxiety, and less pain) almost immediately.

2. DRINK CLEAN WATER

Water is found inside our cells, which is why we need a pure source of water to replenish what our cells and bodies use each day. Anyone who argues that plain tap water is fine needs only to look at Detroit's drinking water travesty to understand the depth of the water issue in our country today. And it's not getting any better, as indicated by the fact that residues of prescription drugs, including opioids, have been found in our water.[109] Even well water should be suspect unless it's been tested and found to be safe. (You can have this testing done by a certified well water testing lab in the state where your well is located.) Today, our natural water supply is woefully full of toxins and void of minerals that are essential to health.

How to make sure your water is clean The ideal drinking water today is filtered house water, which helps eliminate most of the toxins coming through the tap, and/or mineral water in a glass bottle. (This water is filled with natural minerals and none of the toxins found in tap water.) I recommend installing a whole house water filter, along with a tap filter on every faucet from which people drink, as well as a shower and bath filter.A whole house water filter removes sediment, chlorine, fluoride, and heavy metals like lead and aluminum. A tap filter, which improves odor and taste, generally filters out chlorine, pesticides, herbicides, bacteria, parasites, and chemicals like benzene and asbestos. But check each filter for information on exactly what is filtered out, as every filter is different. Keep in mind, however, that when filtering your tap water, you do need to make sure you're also getting enough minerals in your diet (see below), as some filters (like reverse osmosis) not only remove the toxins but also remove essential minerals. In fact, if you are using a reverse osmosis system, I recommend drinking mineral water and using the reverse osmosis water for cooking only.

What you're storing your water in should also be examined. I recommend glass and stainless-steel water bottles to my patients, as plastic bottles have been shown to leach toxins into your drinking water, particularly when there's heat involved. One study showed that hard plastic or polycarbonate bottles can leach BPA, the toxin that can disrupt hormones within the body, into the water. While it didn't matter in the study whether the water was cool or warm, BPA leached significantly faster when boiling water was poured into the plastic.[110] You may think, *I don't pour hot water into my water bottles,* but you may in fact leave your water bottle in a car where water temperature can rise quickly on a hot day. This is why it's best to never drink from a plastic bottle after it's been left in a hot car.

This fact also holds true for the disposable plastic water bottles you buy from a store. One study from the University of Florida found that disposable plastic water bottles stored in a hot car had significantly higher levels of the toxins BPA and antimony (a cancer-causing toxin) than bottles that hadn't been left in the car.[111] And these are only the toxins we know about. There are probably other toxins in plastic bottles we haven't yet discovered that are also health disruptors. The bottom line: make a vow to switch from plastic water bottles to glass or stainless steel to keep your water as clean as possible.

3. GET THE RIGHT NUTRIENTS

Clean farm-to-table eating will help, but sometimes eating all the right foods doesn't necessarily ensure your body gets everything it needs, particularly if you're already deficient in key nutrients. I test all my patients for nutrient deficiencies because without the right vitamins, minerals, fatty acids, proteins, and other nutrients, the body can't tilt the seesaw back in the direction of health.

Nutrients are also critical because they're essential for the development and function of healthy cells. When you don't get enough of the proper nutrients, our cells don't have what they need to do their job properly, particularly if the body is fighting an onslaught of stressors. It's like trying to send an email without a functioning keyboard. It's an impossible task.

When you don't get enough of the proper nutrients, our cells don't have what they need in order to do their job properly, particularly if the body is fighting an onslaught of stressors. It's like trying to send an email without a functioning keyboard. It's an impossible task.

There are several key nutrients our cells and bodies need for optimal health.

• **Essential fatty acids** like omega-6 and omega-3 are a critical part of a healthy body, particularly cellular membranes. Without enough of these healthy fats or too many unhealthy fats, cell membranes can become brittle and/or develop gaps, creating leaks and making it difficult for nutrients to enter cells and waste to move out of cells. If waste can't move out of cells efficiently, cells become toxic. Over time, this toxicity can start to affect cellular DNA. Multiply this by all the cells in the body, and you can begin to see why the seesaw starts to tilt and disease sets in.

Omega-6 and omega-3 fatty acids are likewise critical for the health of the brain and nervous system, namely optimal functioning of brain neurotransmitters, as well as learning, memory, mood, mental clarity, concentration, and focus. (The brain is nearly 60 percent fat and the nervous system is comprised mainly of fat.)

It was scientist Bruce Lipton who likened the cell to a computer, with the cell membrane and its receptors "an organic computer chip." The cell nucleus in his analogy was like the hard drive with DNA-coded software. All the messages that the cell sends to neighboring cells emanate from the membrane, or keyboard. Therefore, when the cell membrane is unstable or "missing keys," the messages being sent out are skewed. This is why I have found that the degree of fatty acid deficit often correlates to the severity of the neurological symptoms. These symptoms include but are not limited to: numbness, tingling, weak hand strength, double vision, "pins and needles" feelings throughout the body, and clumsiness. I describe this imbalance to my patients by explaining that nerves are like copper wires that are missing their protective sheaths or membranes, causing sparks to fly everywhere.

It's no wonder then that children with behavioral problems like ADHD seem to benefit from supplementation with essential fatty acids. Forty-seven percent of children in one study showed an improvement in symptoms after supplementation. In fact, in a new way of thinking about mental health, medical experts have begun to understand that the balance of fatty acids on the cell membrane is related to either mood normalcy or mood disorder. In additional studies, a deficiency of these fatty acids has also been linked with anxiety, dyslexia, dementia, depression, bipolar disorder, and schizophrenia.[112]

What's critical, too, is that you're getting the proper ratio (ideally four to one) of omega-6 to omega-3 fatty acids. If there's not enough intake or too much intake of omega-6 fatty acids (also called linoleic acid) and not enough intake or too much intake of omega-3, then cellular inflammation develops. When you consider that the typical American diet contains, on average, sixteen times more omega-6 fatty acids than omega-3 fatty acids, you can see how vital it is to be mindful of that ratio.[113]

How to get enough Because the body cannot produce essential fatty acids, we must obtain them from food or if needed, from supplements. Healthy dietary sources of omega-6 fatty acids include sunflower seeds (as well as sunflower oil and sunflower seed butter), eggs, organic grass-fed dairy, and chicken and turkey. Healthy sources of omega-3 fatty acids include wild-caught seafood like salmon and sardines, grass-fed beef, nuts like walnuts, flaxseeds and flaxseed oil, and green leafy vegetables.

To break it down even further, it's helpful to understand that there are three types of omega-3 fatty acids: alpha-linolenic acid or ALA (found in nuts, seeds, sunflower oil, and flaxseed oil), eicosapentaenoic acid or EPA (which can be found in marine sources like fish and fish oils), and docosahexaenoic acid or DHA (which can be found in fish and fish oils, as well as in eggs and dairy). There are also linoleic (LA) and gamma-linolenic acid (GLA), both omega-6 fatty acids, which your body also needs.

Each type of fatty acid plays a different role in the body. **ALA** plays a key role in the health of the heart and the blood vessels. **EPA** is key for reducing inflammation in the body and in the brain. **DHA** is necessary for optimal functioning of cellular membranes. **LA** is essential for the health of mitochondria, the powerhouses of each cell responsible for producing cellular energy. **GLA** helps with skin healing and menstrual regularity. If you are supplementing, you want to not only look for one that offers the proper ratio of omega-6 to omega-3 fatty acids, you also want one that offers these additional types, depending on your health concerns. The key with fatty acid supplementation is not to overdo it since too much of one kind will often throw the balance of the others off. We see this in particular today with numerous products (like eggs and snack foods) touting omega-3 fatty acids. When considering these types of foods, it's important to consider what other sources of omega-3 fatty acids you're getting in your diet, since too many omega-3s can be a problem too. Again, balance (that is, a ratio of four omega-6 fatty acids to one omega-3 fatty acid) is key.

One of my favorite ways to naturally "supplement" essential fatty acids is to make a big batch of trail mix on Sundays for the week ahead that contains a healthy balance of fatty acids. I mix in raw, organic nuts (like walnuts, which are high in omega-3 fatty acids) and seeds (like pumpkin seeds, which are high in omega-6 fatty acids), dark chocolate chips, raw coconut flakes, and raisins or goji berries for extra sweetness. I bag it for lunches, soccer meets, and midafternoon snacks, and my kids love it. Again, food is always the best way of supplementing nutrients.

• **Protein** is critical for energy production and repair of DNA (which is stored in a cell's nucleus, the control center of each cell). Every tissue in the body requires protein to maintain structure. Because day-to-day life breaks down our tissues, we need to consume protein to repair and rebuild what's broken. Without enough protein, energy production and energy levels slow down dramatically. This is why I recommend eating a clean, toxin-free source of protein at least once or twice a day depending on how active you are. Athletes may need to eat up to twice as much.

Children also require enough protein for growth, but while they should be receiving more nutrition than adults, instead it is grossly reversed. Not only are children eating less protein than adults, but they are frequently existing on chicken fingers, French fries, and macaroni and cheese. Could you survive on that day after day? The truth is, if parents ate what kids so often eat, we wouldn't be able to get through the day because we'd feel so sluggish. And we wonder why behavioral issues are on the rise. These children don't feel well and act hyper and distractible because their growing bodies and developing brains are starved of key nutrients like protein that they need to properly function.

How to get enough Clean sources of protein include organic beans and legumes, nuts, and seeds. Antibiotic-free meat and pasture-raised eggs are also good. Animals treated with antibiotics breed hard-to-treat super bacteria that are resistant to antibiotics. When animals are treated with antibiotics through their food, not all of the targeted bacteria die. Not only do these animals end up with hard-to-treat super bacteria that are resistant to antibiotics, but those that survive then multiply; when you eat the meat, you consume these bacteria, which can alter your microbiome. Also choose grass-fed beef over grain-fed. Bovines are meant to eat grass. When they do, they produce omega-3 fatty acids in their bodies (which is why grass-fed meat is significantly higher in these fatty acids).[114]

When it comes to seafood, less oily wild fish tends to have fewer toxins like mercury and bacteria than fish that are farm-raised. This is why I recommend wild salmon, halibut, anchovies, sardines, and mackerel. Large fatty fish like swordfish, Chilean sea bass, king mackerel, tuna, and orange roughy tend to be higher in mercury. In addition, wild fish usually have fewer parasites than farm-raised fish because the water they swim in is typically less polluted. (Fish, particularly raw fish, are a common source of parasites that end up in our gut.)

So how much protein do you need? The recommended daily allowance (RDA) for protein is a minimal 0.8 grams per kilogram of body weight. To find this number, multiply your weight in pounds by 0.36. For example, a

140-lb person (140 x .36) would require 50.4 grams of protein according to the RDA. However, that may not even be enough. This RDA is the absolute minimum you need to prevent sickness, not what you need for optimal functioning. (To put this into perspective: one egg has six grams of protein, while three ounces of salmon has seventeen grams.) This is why experts recommend that getting up to twice the RDA in the form of high-quality protein is best for optimal health.[115] I would agree, particularly if you're eating it as part of a healthy farm-to-table diet.

• **Minerals** are the key to unlocking enzymes, which are biological molecules that control the rate of chemical reactions in our cells. As mentioned earlier, enzymes work optimally if a mineral, such as potassium, selenium, sodium, or magnesium, is bound to them. But if there are no minerals, enzymes will find something else to bind to instead, especially toxic heavy metals like aluminum, lead, mercury, and cadmium. Once this happens, the enzymes function very poorly, if at all.

Let's say, for example, that an enzyme binds with mercury. Now we have mercury instead of magnesium in our cells and in our bodies, decreasing brain function and the function of other body systems. The more this happens, the more inflammation, the more fatigue, and the worse a patient feels.

Day by day, our enzymes, throughout every cell in the body, absorb either minerals or heavy metals. It follows, then, that when we eat a mineral-rich diet or take mineral supplements, we give our bodies the chance to support its enzymes with minerals instead of toxic metals. Every day in my practice, I see both children and adults who are so mineral deficient from their diet that they cannot begin to get well until I supplement them for several weeks or months to bring their mineral base back up. Only then can their body begin the process of healing.

Without sufficient levels of key minerals needed for optimal neuro-processing, attention and behavior problems can set in, particularly among children. Growing and developing brains simply don't have what they need to self-regulate. In fact, one of the most catalytic changes in our health today is that our foods are not providing us with enough minerals to keep our bodies well.

How to get enough Swap out your salt shaker. Many people are surprised by the fact that iodized salt isn't healthy for you. It may have small levels of iodine, but it has little else. Pink Himalayan salt, on the other hand, is chock-full of minerals. I recommend using this kind of salt, sold at many stores. In addition, try drinking a mineral water that has high levels of minerals. If you want to supplement, I recommend referring to ConsumerLab.com, which conducts independent research on the best supplements, including mineral supplements.

IODINE: HOW MUCH DOES THE BODY NEED?

The butterfly-shaped thyroid gland, located right below our larynx, works to maintain a proper hormonal balance in the body. It knows what it needs (in this case, iodine), seeks it out in the bloodstream, captures it through cellular receptors, converts it to a hormone, and then stores it for use.

Thyroid hormones are critical for almost every major process in the body, including but not limited to effective functioning of our metabolism (think weight loss or weight gain), growth and development of both tissue and muscle, healthy breasts (low iodine levels can trigger the lumps and bumps characteristic of fibrocystic disease, as well as breast changes that may contribute to cancer), proper brain functioning particularly when it comes to fetal development and infant and childhood brain development, and body temperature. These hormones even influence our enterohepatic circulation. Lack of thyroid hormones in the body contribute to decreased bile flow, which can lead to constipation and the formation of gallstones.

How much iodine, then, is enough? The amount most Americans are currently getting is insufficient. The body cannot make iodine, so we must get it from outside sources. But while most people are aware of the need for common nutrients like calcium and vitamin C, they are not aware of the need for iodine.

This lack of awareness, coupled with the bromide dominance in the body that I mentioned earlier (see page 34), is contributing to mass iodine deficiency in this country. The US Recommended Daily Allowance (RDA) for iodine is currently 150µg (micrograms) per day for anyone age fourteen and older; in pregnant women, it's 220µg per day; and for breastfeeding women, it's 290µg per day.

Before you rush to add iodine to your diet, however, there are some important caveats. The best sources of iodine come from foods like organic grass-fed dairy, organic cage-free eggs, and sea kelp and nori or edible seaweed, not supplements. In fact, in Japan, a country where iodine-rich sea vegetables are a staple of the diet, people are not deficient in this critical trace mineral and, not surprisingly, they also have low rates of endocrine cancers and breast cancer.

This is why I always recommend a food-based multivitamin with a food-based source of iodine, which is more readily absorbed and utilized by the body than a synthetic form of iodine. Two trusted brands that are readily available are MegaFood and New Chapter. For some patients who may require more iodine (levels of which can be checked in both blood and urine), I often recommend supplementing through cooking with seaweed. To do so, put a large kelp leaf (you can buy these dried in grocery stores) in a soup pot while making soup or grains once a week. You can also add kelp leaves to bathwater, as we can absorb iodine through the skin too.

4. EAT FERMENTED FOODS

We need a source of cultured good bacteria in our gut, as these are essential for an optimally functioning microbiome. Replenishing our gut's good bacteria helps to rebalance the microbiota, particularly if someone is on or has been taking antibiotics. Put simply, the greater numbers of healthy bacteria you have in your gut, the less chance harmful bacteria have to survive and thrive. Adding healthy bacteria to the diet is a simple way to treat dysbiosis in both children and adults. Healthy bacteria also ensure a healthy gut–brain axis and optimal brain functioning.

How to replenish the gut's good bacteria Your best bet is to get healthy bacteria from food, which remains the ideal way to get a daily dose. This includes cultured organic dairy products like yogurt and kefir, cultured vegetables like sauerkraut, pickles, kimchi, natto (a Japanese fermented soybean dish), miso, tempeh, and fermented vegetable juice like kombucha. Keep in mind that many of these foods (like kimchi, natto, and kombucha) are an acquired taste, which is why when eating these foods for the first time, I suggest starting with a small amount and trying a food more than once if you didn't care for it the first time. For those who simply don't like these foods or cannot eat them, the next best alternative is to take daily probiotics. Probiotic supplements include healthy bacteria that go by names like *Lactobacillus, Streptococcus thermophilus,* and *Bifidobacterium.* I advise patients who are taking probiotic supplements to rotate the types of probiotics they take every couple of months or so since the gut needs to replenish the hundreds of strains found in it and one single supplement cannot do that.

5. KEEP THE LIVER HEALTHY

One of the most effective ways to keep your liver functioning in optimal health is to limit, as much as possible, your exposure to toxins and to maintain a healthy weight. Eating junk food with artificial ingredients, dyes, and sweeteners (all toxins that the liver has to process) has a direct result on weight and weight gain. The more you eat, the more toxins your liver has to detoxify and the heavier you are. Weight gain and obesity also put a burden on the entire body, including the liver, by triggering a condition called nonalcoholic fatty liver disease. This is one of the fastest growing forms of liver disease, where fat accumulates inside the cells of the liver, taking up about 5–10 percent of the liver's weight and triggering inflammation and scarring/damage to liver tissue.[116] Fatty liver disease is also a trigger for diabetes.

Fatty liver disease is also seen in people who drink too much alcohol, as the alcohol triggers the accumulation of fat cells in the liver. But as obesity levels rise in our country, this disease, which is a precursor to numerous chronic disease conditions, is becoming more rampant and untreated. People with insulin resistance (which is an inability by cells to use the hormone insulin, needed by cells to absorb glucose for energy), high blood sugar, and high levels of fats in the blood are more susceptible to fatty liver disease.

The symptoms of early-stage fatty liver disease are inflammation of the liver, along with common symptoms that may go unrecognized or undiagnosed: fatigue, weakness, loss of weight or appetite, difficulty concentrating, and/or pain in the upper right abdomen where the liver is located. Some people also develop dark-colored patches on the neck or under the arms. Blood tests that measure liver enzyme levels can help diagnose the condition, as can an ultrasound of the liver, which can highlight inflammation.

How to keep your liver in optimal health Eat farm to table and limit your exposure (as much as possible) to toxins in your food, the air, your home, your environment, and your personal care products. It's also important to move your body every day to help boost circulation. Starting your day by drinking water with apple cider vinegar or fresh organic lemon juice can also help keep your liver healthy. (See Your Two-Week Health-Boosting Plan, page 155.) All of these steps help keep your weight in check and your liver and body in balance. Start today to eat healthier and, if you need to, keep track of your food intake so you can drop necessary pounds. Keeping your weight in balance will also prevent type 2 diabetes and other diseases and keep your body healthier overall.

6. RESPECT YOUR IMMUNE SYSTEM

In today's modern society, we're all so anxious to not miss work or school that we force our bodies to recover from illness as quickly as possible. But sometimes the body simply needs to rest and allow itself to recover completely. Our immune system is powerful if we help support it. A fever, which so many people try to suppress with pain killers and fever reducers, is the body's powerful way of fighting a virus or infection.

How to support your immune system Allow your body to be unwell from time to time. The next time you get a fever, avoid taking acetaminophen or ibuprofen and allow the fever to run its course. Letting the body naturally process a fever is the best thing you can do to aid the body during illness. (The only exception to this rule is in small children, where fever must be watched more closely.) Fever is a natural way of cleansing and detoxifying the body—it literally burns up certain unwanted fats, germs, and viruses that congest our tissues and slow down our enterohepatic circulation, ultimately contributing to inflammation. Although this is how the body *should* work, most simply do not today.

Next, slowly reduce your sugar intake, something that's not easy, which is why there are plenty of books written on this very subject. Cutting down on sugar is no easy task and definitely can't be done overnight. It requires time, since sugar addiction can be very strong and cutting it out "cold turkey" can can cause withdrawal symptoms—not unlike a drug withdrawal—like headaches and fatigue. But despite the possible challenges, this is the first step toward a stronger immune system and better health. Start by choosing one time of the day that you typically have cravings for things like cookies, cake, and ice cream and substitute the craving with a piece of fruit or, if necessary, a piece of dark chocolate with a cacao content of 80 percent or higher. These bars tend to have much less sugar and higher antioxidants than the milk chocolate varieties. Then, over time, move onto another meal or snack time. As you start to become more sugar savvy, read food labels to determine how much sugar is in a product and choose foods marked "no added sugar."

A quick tip: If sugar (or cane sugar or fructose) appears in the top three ingredients on a food label, that particular food is laden with sugar and not a good dietary option. Chemical alternatives to sugar, such as sucralose, aspartame, saccharine, xylitol, acesulfame K, and sorbitol are not good options either—you're merely replacing one toxin with another. Better bets include organic honey, maple syrup, and turbinado sugar or "raw" sugar.

7. GET SOME FRESH AIR

Everyone needs more fresh, unpolluted air, particularly if you spend a lot of time indoors, at home or in an office.

How to breathe in cleaner air If this means you have to open your windows more often, then do it. And make it a point to get out in nature more often. Trees help to clean the air, as their leaves help catch and absorb a substantial amount of harmful pollution. In fact, scientists have found that deciduous trees like oak, elm, maple, and birch absorb air pollution nationwide. High Efficiency Particulate Air (HEPA) filters or purifiers at home and at work can also be helpful to clean dust, pollen, mold spores, and animal dander from indoor air. A vacuum with a HEPA filter can also ensure that these indoor air pollutants don't get released back into the air. [117]

8. DETOX EVERY SINGLE DAY

Due to the toxins we're all exposed to daily, each and every person in America today needs to incorporate some simple elements of detoxification into their daily routines to stay healthy. Without sufficient balancers, particularly minerals, toxins can quickly build up in the body. Daily detox options include the following (choose one or two, not all).

• **Break a sweat.** When it comes to sweating, cardiovascular exercise is key. It keeps the body moving, but it also produces sweat, which helps to release toxins from the body. For thousands of years, cultures have used heat to expel toxins from the body for greater health. While we don't need to recreate the Native American sweat lodges to be healthy, we do need the ability to properly vacuate (release or clear out) our bodies to help get rid of the waste we accumulate. If cells aren't able to properly rid themselves of waste, they become toxic. The same thing happens to our bodies on a much larger scale.

 If cells aren't able to properly rid themselves of waste, they become toxic. The same thing happens to our bodies on a much larger scale.

The problem is that we don't allow ourselves to properly vacuate anymore (through sweat and/or through proper bowel movements). We avoid sweat if we can, we take medication to bring down fevers, and we're a culture of the chronically constipated.

How to do it If the exercise you're doing isn't producing sweat, I recommend sitting in a dry heat sauna for ten to fifteen minutes every day. One systematic review of studies found that heavy metal toxins like arsenic, cadmium, lead, and mercury can be released through sweat.[118] This same review of studies shows that up to 20 percent of sweat can include these toxins. What this means is that while you're not sweating everything out all at once, making it a point to sweat every day, along with living a healthy lifestyle, is one step toward keeping your body in balance.

• **Take a detox bath.** If you have an infection, let's say under a fingernail or toenail, one of the easiest ways to treat the swelling and inflammation is to soak that finger or toe in warm water with dissolved Epsom salts. The Epsom salts (magnesium sulfate) literally draw out the pus and infection, helping the finger or toe to heal.

Why this works: both magnesium and sulfate are minerals that are able to be absorbed through the pores or openings of the skin, which triggers a releasing action for the inflammation. Just as sweat is released through the pores when the body heats up during exercise or in a dry-heat sauna, soaking in warm bath water opens the pores and allows more of these minerals to be absorbed and toxins to be released.

Think about this on a greater scale. Magnesium is critical to the detoxification pathways inside our bodies. By absorbing magnesium through the skin, the body is helped to release toxins back out through the skin. Another key part of the detoxification process is the sulfate, which is an easily absorbable form of the mineral sulfur. One of the detoxification pathways in the body is dependent on sulfur. By soaking in Epsom baths, the sulfur is easily absorbed through the skin into the body and then into the bloodstream.

How to do it Add a cup or two of pure Epsom salts to hot water to first dissolve them, then add the solution to warm bath water and soak for about twenty minutes. An Epsom salt detox bath typically works best before bedtime, as the magnesium helps to relax your muscles, enabling you to sleep more soundly.

• **Drink water with apple cider vinegar or fresh, organic lemon juice every morning.** Drinking any water (instead of coffee, tea, or juice) when you first wake up helps to flush the digestive system, but I've found that adding either apple cider vinegar or lemon juice to it helps boost its effect. While vinegar has been a home remedy for a number of conditions since the days of Hippocrates, apple cider vinegar remains an important detoxification tool for our bodies. Raw, unfiltered apple cider vinegar contains something called "the mother" in it, which is healthy bacteria (aka a probiotic) critical for jump-starting a sluggish microbiome. Drinking eight ounces of room temperature water with two teaspoons of apple cider vinegar in the morning before eating seems to help stimulate the liver, the gallbladder, and our entire enterohepatic circulation, which are essential parts of the natural detoxification process in our bodies. I've also found that the natural acids in lemon juice seem to help stimulate digestion.

How to do it Add two teaspoons of raw, unfiltered apple cider vinegar or fresh, organic lemon juice to an eight-ounce glass of pure water every morning and drink it on an empty stomach. You can add a small amount of raw, organic honey to the apple cider vinegar for taste, if necessary. Note that raw, unfiltered apple cider vinegar looks murky and cloudy and is not clear like other vinegars, which through processing have been depleted of their natural enzymes, minerals, nutrients, and bacteria. It also doesn't taste great, but that momentary distaste can be offset by remembering the immense good it's doing for your body.

• **Take herbs that support more efficient detoxification.** Detoxing herbs include artichoke leaf, dandelion leaf, milk thistle seed, rosemary, turmeric

146

root, caper bush root, chicory seed, yarrow, cilantro, and chlorella. Cilantro and chlorella are green supplements that I have found greatly enhance the liver's ability to detoxify heavy metals from our bodies.

How to do it You can find one or a combination of these herbs in herbal teas, but quality is critical when purchasing herbs, be it in teas or in supplement form. Poor quality herbs cannot only be ineffective, which is a waste of money, but can also be harmful. ConsumerLab.com offers a reputable comparison of natural supplements. Incorporating fresh organic herbs like rosemary, cilantro, and turmeric in cooking whenever possible is also a good way to get your daily dose of herbs.

9. TAKE A FOOD-BASED MULTIVITAMIN

Food is the best way for your body to get the nutrients it needs, but even patients with a pristine farm-to-table organic diet are not getting enough nutrients today. Depleted soil no longer has the vitamins and minerals to give to the plants that become our food. This is why supplements, particularly a good multivitamin, become a necessary part of the modern diet.

How to find the right one for you Check the label of your current multivitamin to see the source of its nutrients. It should list specific foods sources like broccoli, kale, carrots, and citrus fruits. If not, the nutrients are most likely synthetic or created in a factory or lab. Synthetic nutritional supplements may cause effects in the body much like medications, which is why it's never a good idea to take a lot of them without medical supervision. This is why I recommend only well-crafted synthetic vitamins and minerals for patients with severe sensitivities or food reactions. For anyone without sensitivities or food reactions, I recommend food-based multivitamins, which are derived from foods and literally crushed into pill form. (Natural food stores have several brands available.) Always follow the dosage instructions on the label or take the quantity prescribed by your physician.

10. GET PLENTY OF B VITAMINS

B vitamins, namely folate (or vitamin B_9), vitamin B_6, and vitamin B_{12}, are crucial nutrients for the body. They support the nervous system, the immune system, proper brain development, red blood cell formation, and the production of cellular DNA. Most people know of folate (or its synthetic version, folic acid, in supplements and fortified food) as the nutrient essential for preventing serious birth defects during pregnancy. But there's more to folate than that. It's also critical for preventing mood disorders, with studies showing that people deficient in B_9 are more susceptible to depression.[119]

Vitamin B_6 is vital for proper nerve functioning and optimal communication between the brain and nervous system. It also plays a key role in the metabolism of carbohydrates, fats, and protein in the body and helps make amino acids (the building blocks of proteins) and mood hormones like serotonin and dopamine, as well as melatonin. What's more, it helps to support immune function and a healthy cardiovascular system, to name just a few of its key roles in the body. Numerous studies have been done on the lack of vitamin B_6 in the body, linking a deficiency to anemia, mood disorders, PMS symptoms, cognitive disorders, neuropathy, diabetes, and more.[120] What this says is that the body absolutely needs enough B_6 to keep its seesaw in balance.

Vitamin B_{12} plays a crucial role in neurological function, too, which is why a deficiency of this nutrient has also been linked to depression and mental fogginess, particularly in children and the elderly.[121] What's more, vitamin B_{12} plays a key part in the production of red blood cells, which supply oxygen to our organs, thereby helping to regulate energy production. Without enough B_{12}, persistent fatigue, unexplained muscle weakness, and lightheadedness can set in.

How to get enough Getting B vitamins from clean food sources is best. Fruits and vegetables, whole grains, and beans are good sources of folate, while poultry, fish, and brightly colored fruits and vegetables like dark leafy greens, oranges, and cantaloupe tend to be good sources of vitamin B_6. Vitamin B_{12} is found in fish, poultry, meat, eggs, and dairy.

If you're not getting enough B vitamins through your foods or you are vegan or a vegetarian, I recommend that you take a food based B-complex vitamin (like those from MegaFood and New Chapter). This is true even if you have a genetic mutation called MTHFR.[122] I test all my patients for this, as having one or both of the mutations (MTHFR C677T or MTHFR A1298C) determines whether or not that person's body can metabolize and absorb folate properly. Those with these mutations do not process synthetic folic acid as well as those who don't have the mutation.

If you don't know your MTHFR status and want to find out, *any* doctor can order this test for a patient through all the major US labs. Once results come back, you can determine whether any old B-complex vitamin will do or whether you need to take a certain kind of folate or B_{12} pertaining to your mutation. Everyone should ask their doctors more about this, since without proper absorption of B vitamins, people are more prone to neurological and mood disorders.

11. BELIEVE IN THE POWER OF YOUR BODY

Your body is capable of amazing things if only given the chance and the key elements it needs. This is why I can't emphasize enough that you *are* capable of being healthy again. You took the first step by picking up this book. By thinking positively about and feeling grateful for the self-healing mechanisms your body is equipped with, you are taking charge of your wellness.

While there is a crisis of health today and while our bodies are being inundated by unhealthy chemicals, toxins, and a food supply that's deficient in key nutrients, there are things *you* can do to balance out the seesaw in your body and get started on the road to recovery for good.

EPILOGUE

New Medicine, Better Results:
Balanced Seesaws = A Nation of Well

Medicine needs to change. It is as simple as that. We are living in a world with a highly myopic view of illness and disease, one in which it's more accepted today to take a lifetime of medication or have surgery than it is to support the natural healing mechanisms within our own bodies. It's more accepted to believe there is something wrong with us rather than paying attention to all the body does that is right. Gone is our intuitive wisdom on what we need for our bodies to be well, and this simply can't go on. Chronic illness is on the rise at a staggering rate and when it comes to health, quality of life is declining. It doesn't have to be this way if we simply listen to what our bodies are telling us.

The body is capable of working in beautiful harmony if all the systems are functioning optimally and if it's given the tools it needs to spontaneously heal. If we listen to our symptoms, each and every one of them, and recognize them as our bodies' cries for help, then we change our perspective on disease and illness. We can also take back power over our health. Skin rashes, belching, gas, chronic pain, sleeplessness, mood swings, behavioral issues, depression, and so much more are all common signs that something is out of balance in the body, that our seesaws are off-kilter. If we quiet these symptoms, the imbalance in the body only becomes worse, with autoimmune diseases like ulcerative colitis and rheumatoid arthritis, heart disease, diabetes, and even cancer on the horizon. In contrast, if we listen to these symptoms and support the body where it's imbalanced, the body and our seesaw will return to balance again. Optimal wellness *is* within our reach. We simply need a better lens with which to see it.

And speaking of putting the power for our health back into our own hands, consider that **the number one tool for health is nutrition**. Diet is what we have 100 percent control over. We decide what we put into our mouths, so we need to "dump the junk," as some would say. This means setting aside any ingredients you can't recognize and embracing the ones you can; eating an abundance of organic produce and whole grains, healthy fats, grass-fed and antibiotic-free proteins, beans and legumes, and wild fish; and drinking plenty of clean mineral water. If you make it a point to eat healthier starting right now, you'll start to notice that pain recedes, you sleep more soundly, you have more energy to do the things you want to do, you feel better, and your skin glows. You'll feel the results of your own seesaw tipping back into balance within days.

The key is to listen. Our bodies speak loudly with symptoms when they're unhappy.

The next step is to supplement your diet with the key balancers I mention in Chapter Five. Consider these the basics for your health: essential fatty acids, a food-based multivitamin, some form of a probiotic (either through cultured or fermented food or a supplement), a B-complex vitamin, and essential minerals. I've talked about why each of these is critical for the optimal functioning of our bodies, but now it's your turn to see what they can do for you.

If you support the body with these important tools and add in daily deep relaxation breathing exercises to calm the vagus nerve and the nervous system, regular exercise, and proper sleep, and have gratitude every day for who you are and what you can accomplish, you will already be way ahead in getting your seesaw back into balance. This is why I've put together, on page 155, a simple two-week actionable plan, with key tips and advice from this book. Yes, some people will need extra help. Certain diseases are entrenched within the body and symptoms may need to be "peeled back" like the layers of an onion to help someone recover from disease. But optimal health is within everyone's reach.

My sincerest hope is that this book will help to start the conversation about what needs to change with our medical paradigm today. We need better definitions of wellness and better diagnostics to help people understand what's really wrong when the standard labs aren't giving us answers. I am learning every day from my patients now and from my patients who have graduated from sickness to wellness. All of my learnings are in this book.

By using the model laid out in these pages, I have been able to return thousands of patients to a better state of health and a happier, more fulfilled quality of life, many with no further treatment needed. This is a goal that can be achieved by most, if not all. I am hopeful that with continued learning, in time we will become a Nation of Well.

Your Two-Week Health-Boosting Plan

Many of my patients ask for a weekly wellness plan to jump-start their health. Disease doesn't start in a matter of weeks, so I never like to promise that any major changes in health, particularly when it comes to the reversal of illness, can take place over a certain period of time. But what can change: bad habits can begin to shift, eating patterns can take on the promise of better health, and our mind-set about what our body is capable of can dramatically change.

Every day of the following plan offers one baby step toward health. Build on each day by incorporating what you've done the day before with your new step toward change. By the end of the fourteen days, you'll have fourteen new healthy steps that will help to transform the way you feel, the amount of energy you have, and how you're sleeping. With this said, if you're on a medication while you're doing this two-week plan, stay on it. You must be under the care of a medical doctor to go off any medicine. And before you start the plan, invest in a water filter pitcher or faucet filter for your drinking water or plan to buy glass-bottled mineral water to drink.

DAY 1

☐ **<u>TODAY</u> wake up and, before you eat, drink an eight-ounce glass of water with two teaspoons of organic apple cider vinegar or the juice of a fresh organic lemon.** The water should be filtered and at room temperature. This will help jump-start your liver and your enterohepatic circulation, critical to your wellness plan.

DAY 2

✓ **Drink your filtered water with apple cider vinegar or fresh, organic lemon juice** first thing in the morning.

☐ **<u>TODAY</u> rethink your food choices.** Give your pantry and fridge a make-over. Go through your food and snacks and read the labels. If anything has ingredients you can't pronounce or you don't know what they are, set them aside to return to the store (if you can), donate to someone in need (if you want), or toss out (if you feel comfortable doing so). If any processed food—including cereal, crackers, chips, granola bars, or other products—contains genetically modified ingredients (typically the case if the product is not organic or doesn't have a non-GMO label), you're better off setting this food aside too. On your next trip to the grocery store, make it a point to read the labels of every product you're buying to be sure you know and can recognize what each of the ingredients are.

A good rule of thumb: anything with more than five or six ingredients is probably not a good option for your health.

Day 3

✓ **Drink your filtered water with apple cider vinegar or fresh, organic lemon juice** first thing in the morning.

✓ **Rethink your food choices** by choosing whole foods and/or foods with six recognizable ingredients or fewer.

☐ **<u>TODAY</u> get at least five (and ideally, seven) servings of brightly colored organic, fiber-rich fruits and vegetables.** Remember, one whole fruit is one serving, while one cup of fruits or vegetables is generally one serving. The exception: two cups of leafy greens is one serving.

Add them to your breakfast eggs, make a smoothie as a snack (e.g., add berries, a handful of spinach, and a banana to almond milk), and bring fresh organic fruits and vegetables to work or eat them on the go. Organic fruits and vegetables make the best snacks. Adding these to your daily diet will help fill you up so you eat fewer processed snacks.

Day 4

✓ **Drink your filtered water with apple cider vinegar or fresh, organic lemon juice** first thing in the morning.

✓ **Rethink your food choices** by choosing whole foods and/or foods with six recognizable ingredients or fewer.

✓ **Be sure to get your five servings of brightly colored organic fruits and vegetables** today, eliminating as many processed snacks as possible.

☐ **<u>TODAY</u> you're going to be sure to incorporate at least twenty to thirty minutes of sweat-inducing activity.** Sweat is the body's natural way of detoxing. It doesn't matter what you do as long as it builds up a sweat. Walk at a fast pace, run, do a cardiovascular machine like an elliptical trainer or treadmill, book a fitness class, or just turn on some music and dance in your living room. Whatever makes you happy will motivate you to do more. And moving forward, mix up your exercise so you don't get bored. If twenty to thirty minutes sounds like a lot, start with just five minutes or less—even one minute is better than none! Then tomorrow or next week, you can try two minutes, then three, and so on. You can also substitute ten to fifteen minutes in a dry-heat sauna if you don't have a chance to exercise. (Be sure to check with your doctor before starting any exercise regimen.)

Day 5

✓ **Drink your filtered water with apple cider vinegar or fresh, organic lemon juice** first thing in the morning.

✓ **Rethink your food choices** by choosing whole foods and/or foods with six recognizable ingredients or fewer.

✓ **Be sure to get at least five servings of brightly colored organic fruits and vegetables** today.

✓ **Make time for twenty to thirty minutes of sweat-inducing activity** or ten to fifteen minutes in a dry-heat sauna.

☐ <u>**TODAY**</u> **turn off your phone, your computer, your TV, and your Wi-Fi at least one hour before going to bed and keep them off all night long.** For those who want to go one step further, turn off all devices in the bedroom that have "blue lights" (see page 117) or put a small napkin or towel over the light to block its emission. Blue lights are particularly disturbing to our pineal gland and significantly reduce the production of melatonin, affecting sleep quality in some people. See if you sleep better tonight and during the rest of this plan.

Day 6

✓ **Drink your filtered water with apple cider vinegar or fresh, organic lemon juice** first thing in the morning.

✓ **Rethink your food choices** by choosing whole foods and/or foods with six recognizable ingredients or fewer.

✓ **Be sure to get at least five servings of brightly colored organic fruits and vegetables** today.

✓ **Make time for twenty to thirty minutes of sweat-inducing activity** or ten to fifteen minutes in a dry-heat sauna.

✓ **Turn off your electronic devices and your Wi-Fi at least one hour before going to bed** and keep them off all night long.

☐ **TODAY you're going to go off nonorganic grains for the rest of this plan.** This includes bread, crackers, and anything else that includes nonorganic grains. When in doubt, check the ingredients label on a product. Take a trip to your grocery store to explore the foods that you may not have noticed before. Don't feel overwhelmed! There are myriad food websites and blogs that offer delicious ways to try organic heritage wheat and organic whole grains like spelt, millet, quinoa, amaranth, and buckwheat. Pinterest is also a great source of healthy whole grain recipes. Some of my favorite websites include *Organic Authority*, *The Organic Kitchen*, *Deliciously Organic*, and *BabyFoodE* for babies and kids.

Day 7

✓ **Drink your filtered water with apple cider vinegar or fresh, organic lemon juice** first thing in the morning.

✓ **Rethink your food choices** by choosing whole foods and/or foods with six recognizable ingredients or fewer.

✓ **Be sure to get at least five servings of brightly colored organic fruits and vegetables** today.

✓ **Make time for twenty to thirty minutes of sweat-inducing activity** or ten to fifteen minutes in a dry-heat sauna.

✓ **Turn off your electronic devices and your Wi-Fi at least one hour before going to bed** and keep them off all night long.

✓ **Continue to avoid all nonorganic grains,** replacing them with organic and/or heritage grains.

☐ **TODAY stop and take a moment to feel grateful for everything your body can do.** This is something easy that you can practice every single day, for one second, one minute, fifteen minutes, or more. As I've mentioned, gratitude is a powerful emotion that can not only put us in a positive state of mind but also has far-reaching effects on our health and self-esteem.

END OF WEEK ONE

Congratulations! You've come this far with these simple changes. You can definitely make it through the next week. Keep going and be sure to keep track of how you're feeling. Do you have more energy? Are you less bloated? Are you sleeping better? Do you feel more mentally clear? There is a chance you might feel worse at first, but keep at it. Big health changes take time but are accomplished by small, consistent steps every day. And whatever you're feeling, take notes so you can refer back to them.

Day 8

✓ **Drink your filtered water with apple cider vinegar or fresh, organic lemon juice** first thing in the morning.

✓ **Rethink your food choices** by choosing whole foods and/or foods with six recognizable ingredients or fewer.

✓ **Be sure to get at least five servings of brightly colored organic fruits and vegetables** today. <u>This week, though, see if you can increase your intake to a minimum of seven servings daily.</u>

✓ **Make time for twenty to thirty minutes of sweat-inducing activity** or ten to fifteen minutes in a dry-heat sauna.

✓ **Turn off your electronic devices and your Wi-Fi at least one hour before going to bed** and keep them off all night long.

✓ **Continue to avoid all nonorganic grains,** replacing them with organic and/or heritage grains.

✓ **Take a moment to feel grateful** for everything your body can do.

☐ **TODAY you're going to give your household cleaners a makeover, swapping out chemical cleaners for natural, botanical-based ones.** This includes everything from your dishwashing and laundry detergents to your floor and window cleaners. While I admit bleach-based cleansers are hard to give up, the fumes they give off are toxic. Exposure should be minimized to only the toughest spots, like the bathroom. Try swapping these out for chlorine-free formulas that contain a mix of hydrogen peroxide, lemon juice, baking soda, and/or vinegar for the majority of the house.

Day 9

✓ **Drink your filtered water with apple cider vinegar or fresh, organic lemon juice** first thing in the morning.

✓ **Rethink your food choices** by choosing whole foods and/or foods with six recognizable ingredients or fewer.

✓ **Be sure to get five to seven servings of brightly colored organic fruits and vegetables** today.

✓ **Make time for twenty to thirty minutes of sweat-inducing activity** or ten to fifteen minutes in a dry-heat sauna.

✓ **Turn off your electronic devices and your Wi-Fi at least one hour before going to bed** and keep them off all night long.

✓ **Continue to avoid all nonorganic grains,** replacing them with organic and/or heritage grains.

✓ **Take a moment to feel grateful** for everything your body can do.

✓ **Use natural, botanical-based household cleaners** instead of chemical-laden ones.

☐ **TODAY you're going to incorporate deep, diaphragmatic breathing, or what's sometimes called the 4-7-8 breathing exercise, into your daily routine**. I learned about the 4-7-8 breathing technique from Dr. Weil, which I now share with my patients. You choose the time and place, but you want to start by placing your tongue behind your upper front teeth. Keep it there throughout the entire breathing exercise. Close your mouth and inhale slowly to a count of 4. Then hold your breath for a count of 7 before exhaling completely through your mouth. Make a "whoosh" sound to the count of 8 while you're exhaling. As you're breathing in, visualize yourself drawing in air through your toes, up through your body, deep into your lungs, and into your chest. Repeat this at least four or five times, breathing in deeply and breathing out slowly. Be sure to take account of how you feel after doing this. Moving forward, incorporate this into your day whenever you're feeling stressed (e.g., sitting in traffic or before a big meeting) or before bed to help you sleep. But be sure to do it at least once a day.

Day 10

✓ **Drink your filtered water with apple cider vinegar or fresh, organic lemon juice** first thing in the morning.

✓ **Rethink your food choices** by choosing whole foods and/or foods with six recognizable ingredients or fewer.

✓ **Be sure to get five to seven servings of brightly colored organic fruits and vegetables** today.

✓ **Make time for twenty to thirty minutes of sweat-inducing activity** or ten to fifteen minutes in a dry-heat sauna.

✓ **Turn off your electronic devices and your Wi-Fi at least one hour before going to bed** and keep them off all night long.

✓ **Continue to avoid all nonorganic grains,** replacing them with organic and/or heritage grains.

✓ **Take a moment to feel grateful** for everything your body can do.

✓ **Use natural, botanical-based household cleaners** instead of chemical-laden ones.

✓ **Incorporate deep, diaphragmatic breathing into your daily routine** for at least four or five breaths.

☐ **TODAY you're going to add a supplement to your daily routine.** You're going to buy an organic or non-GMO food-based multivitamin and begin to take it every day. Food-based multivitamins are ones that are made from real fruits and vegetables, which are the best sources of the nutrients our body needs. Be sure your multivitamin contains minerals, or take your vitamins with mineral water. Always take the recommended daily amount every day moving forward. You're also going to add probiotics to your diet, either through fermented foods like yogurt, sauerkraut, kefir, pickles, kombucha, or kimchi that you'll eat daily, or through a probiotic supplement with at least 25 to 50 billion CFUs (colony-forming units), a measure of the healthy bacteria in the probiotic.

Day 11

✓ **Drink your filtered water with apple cider vinegar or fresh, organic lemon juice** first thing in the morning.

✓ **Rethink your food choices** by choosing whole foods and/or foods with six recognizable ingredients or fewer.

✓ **Be sure to get five to seven servings of brightly colored organic fruits and vegetables** today.

✓ **Make time for twenty to thirty minutes of sweat-inducing activity** or ten to fifteen minutes in a dry-heat sauna.

✓ **Turn off your electronic devices and your Wi-Fi at least one hour before going to bed** and keep them off all night long.

✓ **Continue to avoid all nonorganic grains,** replacing them with organic and/or heritage grains.

✓ **Take a moment to feel grateful** for everything your body can do.

✓ **Use natural, botanical-based household cleaners** instead of chemical-laden ones.

✓ **Incorporate deep, diaphragmatic breathing into your daily routine** for at least four or five breaths.

✓ **Take your food-based multivitamin and probiotics** today.

☐ **TODAY you're going to assess the personal care products you use on your face and/or body.** This includes body washes, shampoos, conditioners and hairstyling products; facial washes and creams; nail polish; perfume/cologne; sunscreen; and makeup. I want you to look up the ingredients, either on the label or online, and set aside any products that contain the toxins phthalates, parabens, and triclosan. You also want to avoid any active chemical ingredients in sunscreens other than zinc oxide and titanium dioxide. If there are any ingredients you don't recognize, you can look them up online in the Environmental Working Group's Skin Deep Cosmetics Database or use their Healthy Living app. They list ingredients' potential toxicity, along with reasons why they're toxic. Remember that your skin is one of the largest organs in your body. What you put on it is absorbed into the body and will have to be processed by the liver in the same way as the foods you eat. This is why I often say, *Put on your skin only what you would eat.* Once you've done this, begin to swap in products that are made from less toxic ingredients and essential oil–based (or no) fragrances.

Day 12

✓ **Drink your filtered water with apple cider vinegar or fresh, organic lemon juice** first thing in the morning.

✓ **Rethink your food choices** by choosing whole foods and/or foods with six recognizable ingredients or fewer.

✓ **Be sure to get five to seven servings of brightly colored organic fruits and vegetables** today.

✓ **Make time for twenty to thirty minutes of sweat-inducing activity** or ten to fifteen minutes in a dry-heat sauna.

✓ **Turn off your electronic devices and your Wi-Fi at least one hour before going to bed** and keep them off all night long.

✓ **Continue to avoid all nonorganic grains,** replacing them with organic and/or heritage grains.

✓ **Take a moment to feel grateful** for everything your body can do.

✓ **Use natural, botanical-based household cleaners** instead of chemical-laden ones.

✓ **Incorporate deep, diaphragmatic breathing into your daily routine** for at least four or five breaths.

✓ **Take your food-based multivitamin and probiotics** today.

✓ **Start to use fewer (or no) toxic personal care products**.

☐ **<u>TODAY</u> you're going to resolve to purchase only high-quality proteins.** This includes grass-fed antibiotic-free beef, pasture-raised chickens and eggs, and wild-caught fish. Organic beans and legumes are also good vegetarian sources of protein. These may all be pricier, but there are frequently deals on clean proteins at local stores. You can buy in bulk when the prices are better and freeze, thawing only what you need for your meals.

Day 13

✓ **Drink your filtered water with apple cider vinegar or fresh, organic lemon juice** first thing in the morning.

✓ **Rethink your food choices** by choosing whole foods and/or foods with six recognizable ingredients or fewer.

✓ **Be sure to get five to seven servings of brightly colored organic fruits and vegetables** today.

✓ **Make time for twenty to thirty minutes of sweat-inducing activity** or ten to fifteen minutes in a dry-heat sauna.

✓ **Turn off your electronic devices and your Wi-Fi at least one hour before going to bed** and keep them off all night long.

✓ **Continue to avoid all nonorganic grains,** replacing them with organic and/or heritage grains.

✓ **Take a moment to feel grateful** for everything your body can do.

✓ **Use natural, botanical-based household cleaners** instead of chemical-laden ones.

✓ **Incorporate deep, diaphragmatic breathing into your daily routine** for at least four or five breaths.

✓ **Take your food-based multivitamin and probiotics** today.

✓ **Start to use fewer (or no) toxic personal care products.**

✓ **Eat high-quality clean proteins.**

☐ **<u>TODAY</u> you're going to start to reduce the sugar you're eating.** You should be consuming less processed sugar already by eating your seven servings of fruits and vegetables a day, but if you find you're still addicted to sweets, you're going to start giving your taste buds a makeover. First, you want to make sure you get rid of any sugar substitutes. These include chemical sweeteners like aspartame and those little colored packets. Patients often ask me about stevia, extracted from the stevia plant. While stevia does not have the concerns that some of the artificial sweeteners do, it is much sweeter than sugar so again, moderation is key. If you do use stevia, look for the highly purified *organic* form of stevia known as Rebiana or Reb A.

If you're drinking diet drinks, you'll want to replace them with unsweetened black or herbal teas or water naturally flavored with organic lemons, cucumbers, mint, or berries. Take stock of any other sources of sugar in your diet, including hidden sources of sugar in your morning oatmeal, in your nut butters, in your condiments, or in your yogurt and other dairy products. You want to keep your daily sugar intake to a minimum. This is not to say you can never have sugar. Just cut down on your daily intake. And when it comes to the sugar you do eat, make it natural sources like organic honey, maple syrup, and/or raw or turbinado sugar.

Keep in mind that cutting out sugar in the beginning is hard, but after a week or so, your taste buds adjust and you don't crave sugar anymore. At this point, the juicy taste of fresh fruit often becomes enough to satisfy your sweet cravings!

Day 14

✓ **Drink your filtered water with apple cider vinegar or fresh, organic lemon juice** first thing in the morning.

✓ **Rethink your food choices** by choosing whole foods and/or foods with six recognizable ingredients or fewer.

✓ **Be sure to get five to seven servings of brightly colored organic fruits and vegetables** today.

✓ **Make time for twenty to thirty minutes of sweat-inducing activity** or ten to fifteen minutes in a dry-heat sauna.

✓ **Turn off your electronic devices and your Wi-Fi at least one hour before going to bed** and keep them off all night long.

✓ **Continue to avoid all nonorganic grains,** replacing them with organic and/or heritage grains.

✓ **Take a moment to feel grateful** for everything your body can do.

✓ **Use natural, botanical-based household cleaners** instead of chemical-laden ones.

✓ **Incorporate deep, diaphragmatic breathing into your daily routine** for at least four or five breaths.

✓ **Take your food-based multivitamin and probiotics** today.

✓ **Start to use fewer (or no) toxic personal care products.**

✓ **Eat high-quality clean proteins**.

✓ **Reduce your intake of sugar** and sugar substitutes.

☐ **<u>TODAY</u> you're going to be sure that you're eating only organic, grass-fed dairy products moving forward.** This includes milk, yogurt, cheese, and ice cream. You can also swap out dairy products for organic nondairy options like almond milk or coconut milk products. Many people are sensitive to the whey in milk products, which can be a trigger for bloating, digestive upset, and even headaches.

Even though this is the last day of the two-week plan, this is something you can try moving forward for two more weeks to see if you notice any changes in your health or any symptoms you've been experiencing. If you find that you feel better after this swap, make it a permanent part of your get-healthy lifestyle moving forward.

YOU DID IT!

Congratulations! You've just put into place some of the most important health habits. These will all make a difference in how you're feeling. But more than that, you've taken your health into your own hands and seen firsthand how the simplest changes in our daily lives can make a difference in how we feel every day. It doesn't always require a prescription to feel better. Instead, it takes daily changes to put our bodies on the path to health and to recover wellness. This is something that each and every one of us has the power to accomplish.

But don't stop here. Continue putting these daily changes into practice every day moving forward and see if any symptoms you currently have eventually subside. Your health can only benefit from here.

ACKNOWLEDGMENTS

I feel so incredibly blessed to be able to intersect with the lives of my thousands of patients. It is because of them and their journeys that I have learned how the body really works, making this book possible. Many have recovered their health completely as a result, and all have provided the learnings for me that went on to help others even more. I thank all of my patients. Each one has been part of my beautiful journey to help guide health, and hopefully in time, *healthcare,* to a better place. And through it all, I have had the extreme blessing of my supportive, loving husband and three beautiful sons, along with my loving family. Without their support and love at home, I would not have found the strength to do my work.

Joel Gedroic Thank you to my husband for being my rock.

Logan, Colton, and Rex Gedroic Thank you to my three beautiful sons for being angels on earth. God's true light shines in all three of you. You have already taught me more than I can ever teach you. Thank you.

Joan Wegman Goldberg Thank you to my mother, who always believed in me.

Victoria Profeta Thank you to my sister for being my best friend and true champion. You have always helped me believe in myself even when I didn't.

Gary Goldberg Thank you for your enduring love and for always being there for me.

Theresa Myers Thank you for being my role model.

Paul Profeta Thank you for teaching me to dream big and never give up.

Ray Chambers Thank you for your support and inspiration. Your light shines ever bright and touches many.

Danny Wegman Thank you for your belief in me.

Colleen Wegman Thank you for our "walks." Each year, your inspiration helps me push the ball further.

Michael Cooper Thank you for your energy and connection.

Nancy, Deirdra, Eva, and TC Thank you for our friendship, which continues to endure for all time.

All of my extended family Thank you for the roots of true love.

Dr. Patricia Kane Thank you for the hours and hours of research shared, your teachings, and your vision.

Dr. Damien Downing Thank you for teaching me epigenetics in clinical medicine.

Drs. Meinrad Milz and *Katrin Beiber* Thank you for teaching me how true healing in the body begins and for continuing to be close friends.

Dr. Ann Corson Thank you for starting me on this path. Your teachings I hold dear.

Dr. Richard Horowitz Thank you for teaching me a new way of looking at disease.

Dr. Roger Granet I am forever grateful for your compassion. The door had closed, but you opened a window.

Dr. Mehmet Oz Your passion was an inspiration. Thank you for exciting me about pursuing surgery.

Dr. Andrew Weil Thank you for opening my eyes to a whole new medical paradigm.

Monique Bureau For opening me up to see so much more.

Fred Profeta Sr. You are with me all the time.

Judy Loring Thank you for being my dear friend and for all that you have taught me.

Susan McCamish Thank you for being my dear friend and kindred in journey.

The GMI staff It takes a village of love to heal the sick. Thank you all for being part of the team.

Judy Dreskin Thank you for your wonderful contribution to this book.

Valerie Latona Without your time and attention, my passion to reach others would not be a reality.

With extreme gratitude,
Kristine Gedroic, MD

Resources

INTRODUCTION

1   Van Cleave, J., S.L. Gortmaker, and J.M. Perrin. "Dynamics of Childhood Obesity and Chronic Health Conditions Among Children and Youth." *JAMA* 303, no 7 (February 17, 2010): 623–30. https://www.ncbi.nlm.nih.gov/pmc/articles/PMC3319320/.

2   Oaklander, Mandy. "New Hope for Depression." *Time,* August 7, 2017. http://time.com/4876098/new-hope-for-depression/.

CHAPTER ONE
Chronic Sickness on the Rise, Despite Medical Advances

3   Ward, B.W., J.S. Schiller, and R.A. Goodman. "Multiple Chronic Conditions Among US Adults: a 2012 Update." *Preventing Chronic Disease* 2014;11:130389. DOI: http://dx.doi.org/10.5888/pcd11.130389. Dennis, Brady. "Nearly 60 Percent of Americans—the Highest Ever—Are Taking Prescription Drugs." *The Washington Post.* November 3, 2015. https://www.washingtonpost.com/news/to-your-health/wp/2015/11/03/more-americans-than-ever-are-taking-prescription-drugs/?utm_term=.6d3b4a8c1e66.

4   "Health: United States 2016 with Chartbook on Long-Term Trends in Health." pp. 23, 293. Accessed January 13, 2018. https://www.cdc.gov/nchs/data/hus/hus16.pdf#079. "Therapeutic Drug Use." National Center for Health Statistics. Accessed September 15, 2018. https://www.cdc.gov/nchs/fastats/drug-use-therapeutic.htm

5   "CDC: US Deaths from Heart Disease, Cancer on the Rise." *American Heart Association News.* Accessed October 8, 2017. https://www.heart.org/

en/news/2018/07/17/cdc-us-deaths-from-heart-disease-cancer-on-the-rise. Health: United States 2016 with Chartbook on Long-Term Trends in Health." Add "Accessed October 8, 2017. https://www.cdc.gov/nchs/data/hus/hus16. pdf#019; "Leading Causes of Death." Centers for Disease Control and Prevention, NCHS FastStats website. Accessed June 5, 2016. http://www. cdc.gov/nchs/fastats/leading-causes-of-death.htm. Nichols, Hannah. "The Top 10 Leading Causes of Death in the United States." *Medical News Today.* February 23, 2017. https://www.medicalnewstoday.com/articles/282929.php. "Autoimmune Disease Statistics." American Autoimmune Related Diseases Association, Inc. Accessed January 13, 2018. https://www.aarda.org/news-information/statistics/. Lerner, Aaron, Patricia Jermemais, and Torsten Matthias. "The World Incidence and Prevalence of Autoimmune Disease Is Increasing." *International Journal of Celiac Disease* 3, no 4 (2015): 151–55. http://pubs.sciepub.com/ijcd/3/4/8/.

6   Van Cleave, Jeanne, MD, Steven L. Gortmaker, PhD, and James M. Perrin, MD. "Dynamics of Obesity and Chronic Health Conditions Among Children and Youth." *JAMA* 303, no 7 (Feb. 17, 2010): 623–30. https://jamanetwork. com/journals/jama/fullarticle/185391.

7   Eveleth, Rose. "There Are 37.2 Trillion Cells in Your Body." *Smithsonian. com.* October 24, 2013. http://www.smithsonianmag.com/smart-news/ there-are-372-trillion-cells-in-your-body-4941473/.

8   "Size of the Nanoscale." *Nanotechnology 101.* United States National Nanotechnology Initiative. Accessed June 18, 2018. https://www.nano.gov/ nanotech-101/what/nano-size.

CHAPTER TWO
The Evolution of Medicine: How We Got Where We Are Today

9   Cohen, Jennie. "A Brief History of Bloodletting." History in the Headlines. *History* (May 30, 2012). https://www.history.com/news/a-brief-history-of-bloodletting.

10   "Life in the 1700s: Coping with Disease." National Park Service, US Department of the Interior, Guilford Courthouse, National Military Park. Accessed May 13, 2017. https://www.nps.gov/guco/planyourvisit/upload/ Diseases.pdf.

11   Petrovska, Biljana Bauer. "Historical Review of Medicinal Plants' Usage." *Pharmacognosy Review* 6, no 11 (Jan–Jun 2012): 1–5. https://www.

ncbi.nlm.nih.gov/pmc/articles/PMC3358962/. "Fernleaf, Biscuitroot; Lomatium Dissectum." *Plant Guide,* United States Department of Agriculture. Accessed January 13, 2018. https://www.fs.fed.us/rm/pubs_other/rmrs_2011_tilley_d002.pdf. "Lomatium." *Encyclopedia.com.* Accessed January 13, 2018. http://www.encyclopedia.com/medicine/encyclopedias-almanacs-transcripts-and-maps/lomatium.

12 Oneill, Therese. "8 Drugs That Exist in Nature." *The Week* (May 29, 2013). http://theweek.com/articles/464010/8-drugs-that-exist-nature. Wu, Jessica. "Where Does Medicine Come From?" *Science in the News.* Harvard University (June 5, 2011). http://sitn.hms.harvard.edu/flash/2011/where-does-medicine-come-from/.

13 Deziel, Chris. "The Effects of Industrial Smog." *Sciencing* (April 25, 2017). http://sciencing.com/effects-industrial-smog-8152.html.

14 Brugge, Doug, John L. Durant, and Christine Rioux. "Near-Highway Pollutants in Motor Vehicle Exhaust: A Review of Epidemiologic Evidence of Cardiac and Pulmonary Health Risks." *Environmental Health* (Aug. 9, 2007). https://ehjournal.biomedcentral.com/articles/10.1186/1476-069X-6-23.

15 "Lead Poisoning and Health." *Media Center Fact Sheet,* World Health Organization (August 2017). http://www.who.int/mediacentre/factsheets/fs379/en/.

16 "Bacillus Thuringiensis: Synthetic Pesticides." University of California San Diego. Accessed July 18, 2017. http://www.bt.ucsd.edu/synthetic_pesticide.html.

17 DeJesus, Erin. "A Brief History of Spam, an American Meat Icon." Eater.com. July 9, 2014. https://www.eater.com/2014/7/9/6191681/a-brief-history-of-spam-an-american-meat-icon.

18 Schlosser, Eric. "Excerpt: Fast Food Nation." *PBS.* Accessed July 18, 2017. http://www.pbs.org/pov/foodinc/excerpt-fast-food-nation/3/.

19 Leung, Angela M., Lewis E. Braverman, and Elizabeth N. Pearce. "History of US Iodine Fortification and Supplementation." *Nutrients* 4, no 11 (Nov. 4, 2012): 1740–46. https://www.ncbi.nlm.nih.gov/pmc/articles/PMC3509517/.

20 Smyth, Peter, P.A. "The Thyroid, Iodine, and Breast Cancer." *Breast Cancer Research* 5, no 5 (2003): 235–38. https://www.ncbi.nlm.nih.gov/pmc/articles/PMC314438/. Kilbane, M.T., R.A. Ajjan, A.P. Weetman, et al. "Tissue Iodine Content and Serum Mediated 125I Uptake Blocking Activity in Breast Cancer." *The Journal of Clinical Endocrinology and Metabolism* 85

(2000): 1245–50. https://www.ncbi.nlm.nih.gov/pubmed/10720070. Gulaboglu, Mine, Leyla Yildiz, Mustufa Gul, et al. "Blood and Urine Iodine Levels in Patients with Gastric Cancer." *Biological Trace Element Research* 113, no 3 (December 2016): 261–71. https://www.researchgate. net/publication/6605730_Blood_and_Urine_Iodine_Levels_in_Patients_ with_Gastric_Cancer. Rappaport, Jay. "Changes in Dietary Iodine Explains Increasing Incidence of Breast Cancer with Distant Involvement in Young Women." *Journal of Cancer* 8, no 2 (2017): 174–77. https://www.ncbi. nlm.nih.gov/pmc/articles/PMC5327366/. Hollowell, J.G., N.H. Staehling, W.H. Hannon, et al. "Iodine Nutrition in the United States. Trends and Public Health Implications: Iodine Excretion Data from National Health and Nutrition Examination Surveys I and III (1971–1974 and 1988–1994)." *Journal of Clinical Endocrinology and Metabolism* 83, no 10 (October 1998): 2401–8. https://www.ncbi.nlm.nih.gov/pubmed/9768638.

21 Hippocrates, *On Forecasting Diseases*, as seen in *The History Learning Site*. Accessed May 15, 2017. http://www.historylearningsite. co.uk/a-history-of-medicine/hippocrates/.

CHAPTER THREE
How Do We Stay Healthy? Optimizing Our Inner Ecosystem

22 Wolchover, Natalie, "Your Body Harbors Pounds of Microbes, Study Reveals." LiveScience. June 15, 2012. https://www.livescience. com/34004-microbes-human-body.html. Statt, Nick. "Fact: You Carry Around Enough Bacteria to Fill a Large Soup Can." Popular Science. September 12, 2013. https://www.popsci.com/science/article/2011-09/ fyi-how-much-bacteria-do-people-carry-around.

23 Nash, A.K., T.A. Auchtung, M.C. Wong, et al. "The Gut Mycobiome of the Human Microbiome Project Healthy Cohort." *Microbiome* 5, no 1 (November 25, 2017): 153. https://www.ncbi.nlm.nih.gov/ pubmed/29178920. Bizzell, Erica. "The Mycobiome, Fungal Dysbiosis, and Health in the Gut." *Microbial Sciences* 12 (December 22, 2017): 52. https://www.asm.org/Articles/2017/December/the-mycobiome-fungal- dysbiosis-and-health-in-the-g. Cui, Lijia, Alison Morris, and Elodie Ghedin. "The Human Mycobiome in Health and Disease." *Genome Medicine* 5 (July 30, 2013): 63. https://genomemedicine.biomedcentral.com/ articles/10.1186/gm467. Hager, Christopher, and Mahmoud A. Ghannoum. "The Mycobiome: Role in Health and Disease, and as a Potential Probiotic

Target in Gastrointestinal Disease." *Digestive and Liver Disease* 49, no 11 (November 2017): 1171–76. https://www.dldjournalonline.com/article/ S1590-8658(17)31015-0/fulltext.

24 Neu, Josef, MD, and Jona Rushing, MD. "Cesarean Versus Vaginal Delivery: Long-Term Infant Outcomes and the Hygiene Hypothesis." *Clinics in Perinatology* 38, no 2 (June 2011): 321–31. https://www.ncbi.nlm.nih.gov/ pmc/articles/PMC3110651/. Dominguez-Bello, Maria G., Kassandra M. De Jesus-Laboy, and Nan Shen, et al. "Partial Restoration of the Microbiota of Cesarean-Born Infants Via Vaginal Microbial Transfer." *Nature Medicine* 22 (February 1, 2016): 250–53. https://www.nature.com/articles/ nm.4039#auth-2.

25 Koch, Meghan A., Gabrielle L. Reiner, and Kyler A. Lugo, et al. "Maternal IgG and IgA Antibodies Dampen Mucosal T Helper Cell Responses in Early Life." *Cell* 165, no 4 (May 2016): 827–41. http://www.cell.com/cell/ fulltext/S0092-8674(16)30500-1. Mueller, Noel T., Elizabeth Bakacs, Joan Combellick, et al. "The Infant Microbiome Development: Mom Matters." *Trends in Molecular Medicine* 21, no 2 (Feb. 2015): 109–17. https://www.ncbi. nlm.nih.gov/pmc/articles/PMC4464665/. Azad, Meghan, Theodore Konya, Heather Maughan, et al. "Gut Microbiota of Healthy Canadian Infants: Profiles by Mode of Delivery and Infant Diet at 4 Months." *CMAJ* (Feb. 11, 2013). http://www.cmaj.ca/content/early/2013/02/11/cmaj.121189.

26 "Diversifying Your Diet May Make Your Gut Healthier." *ScienceDaily.* Institute of Food Technologists. July 14, 2015. https://www.sciencedaily. com/releases/2015/07/150714142231.htm?utm_source=feedburner&utm_ medium=email&utm_campaign=Feed%3A+sciencedaily%2Ftop_ news%2Ftop_health+%28ScienceDaily%3A+Top+Health+News%29.

27 Feltman, Rachel. "The Gut's Microbiome Changes Rapidly with Diet." *Scientific American.* December 14, 2014. https://www.scientificamerican. com/article/the-guts-microbiome-changes-diet/. Sokolowska, Milena, Remo Frei, Nonhlanhla Lunjani, et al. "Microbiome and Asthma." *Asthma Research and Practice* 4, no 1 (January 5, 2018). https://asthmarp. biomedcentral.com/articles/10.1186/s40733-017-0037-y. Stiemsma, Leah T. and Stuart T. Turvey. "Asthma and the Microbiome: Defining the Critical Window in Early Life." *Allergy, Asthma, and Clinical Immunology* 13, no 3 (January 6, 2017). https://www.ncbi.nlm.nih.gov/pmc/articles/PMC5217603/. Chung, Kian Fan. "Airway Microbial Dysbiosis in Asthmatic Patients: A Target for Prevention and Treatment?" *The Journal of Allergy and Clinical*

Immunology 139, no 4 (April 2017): 1071–81. https://www.jacionline.org/article/S0091-6749(17)30317-2/fulltext.

28 Chase, John, Jennifer Fouquier, Mahnaz Zare, et al. "Geography and Location Are the Primary Drivers of Office Microbiome Composition." *MSystems*, 2016 DOI; http://msystems.asm.org/content/1/2/e00022-16.

29 Wang, Z.K., Y.S. Yang, A.T. Stefka, et al. "Review Article: Fungal Microbiota and Digestive Diseases." *AP&T* 39, no 8 (April 2014): 751–66. https://onlinelibrary.wiley.com/doi/full/10.1111/apt.12665.

30 Tchounwou, Paul B., Clement G. Yedjou, Anita K. Patlolla, et al. "Heavy Metals Toxicity and the Environment." Experienta. Supplementum, no 101 (2012): 133–64. https://www.ncbi.nlm.nih.gov/pmc/articles/PMC4144270/. Breton, Jérôme, Sébastien Massart, Peter Vandamme, et al. "Ecotoxicology Inside the Gut: Impact of Heavy Metals on the Mouse Microbiome." *BMC Pharmacology & Toxicology* (December 11, 2013). https://bmcpharmacol-toxicol.biomedcentral.com/articles/10.1186/2050-6511-14-62. "Persistent Organic Pollutants: A Global Issue, A Global Response." International Cooperation, United States Environmental Protection Agency. Accessed January 13, 2018. https://www.epa.gov/international-cooperation/persistent-organic-pollutants-global-issue-global-response.

31 Samsel, Anthony, and Stephanie Seneff. "Glyphosate Pathways to Modern Diseases V: Amino Acid Analogue of Glycine in Diverse Proteins." *Journal of Biological Physics and Chemistry* 16 (June 2016): 9–46. https://www.researchgate.net/publication/305318376_Glyphosate_pathways_to_modern_diseases_V_Amino_acid_analogue_of_glycine_in_diverse_proteins. Samsel, Anthony, and Stephanie Seneff. "Glyphosate, Pathways to Modern Diseases IV: Cancer and Related Pathologies." *Journal of Biological Physics and Chemistry* 15, no 3 (January 2015): 121–59. https://www.researchgate.net/publication/283490944_Glyphosate_pathways_to_modern_diseases_IV_cancer_and_related_pathologies. "40 CFR 180.364—Glyphosate; Tolerances for Residues." Legal Information Institute, Cornell Law School. Accessed April 23, 2018. https://www.law.cornell.edu/cfr/text/40/180.364?qt-ecfrmaster=0#qt-ecfrmaster. "Adoption of Genetically Engineered Crops in the U.S." USDA Economic Research Service (2015). https://www.ers.usda.gov/data-products/adoption-of-genetically-engineered-crops-in-the-us.aspx. "Glyphosate: Unsafe on Any Plate." Food Democracy Now! and The Detox Project. Accessed April 23, 2018. https://s3.amazonaws.com/media.fooddemocracynow.org/images/FDN_Glyphosate_FoodTesting_Report_p2016.pdf.

32 "Childhood Obesity Facts." Centers for Disease Control and Prevention. Accessed February 12, 2018. https://www.cdc.gov/obesity/data/childhood. html.

33 Woodmansey, E.J. "Intestinal Bacteria and Ageing." *Journal of Applied Microbiology* 102, no 5 (April 19, 2007): 1178–86. http://onlinelibrary.wiley. com/doi/10.1111/j.1365-2672.2007.03400.x/full. Conlon, Michael A., and Anthony R. Bird. "The Impact of Diet and Lifestyle on Gut Microbiota and Human Health." *Nutrients* 7, no 1 (January 2015): 17–44. https://www.ncbi. nlm.nih.gov/pmc/articles/PMC4303825/.

34 Bailey, M.T., S.E. Dowd, J.D. Galley, et al. "Exposure to a Social Stressor Alters the Structure of the Intestinal Microbiota: Implications for Stressor-Induced Immunomodulation." *Brain, Behavior, and Immunity* 25, no 3 (March 2011): 397–407. https://www.ncbi.nlm.nih.gov/pubmed/21040780. Foster, Jane A., Linda Rinaman, and John F. Cryan. "Stress and the Gut-Brain Axis: Regulation by the Gut Microbiome." *Neurobiology of Stress* 7 (December 2017): 124–36. https://www.sciencedirect.com/science/article/pii/S2352289516300509.

35 Ridaura, Vanessa K., Jeremiah J. Faith, Federico E. Rey, et al. "Gut Microbiota from Twins Discordant for Obesity Modulate Metabolism in Mice." *Science* 341, no 6150 (September 2013). http://science.sciencemag.org/content/341/6150/1241214.

36 Round, J.L., and S.K. Mazmanian. "The Gut Microbiota Shapes Intestinal Immune Responses During Health and Disease." *Nature Reviews. Immunology* 9, no 5 (May 2009): 313–23. https://www.ncbi.nlm.nih. gov/pubmed/19343057/; Eddy, K.V.R., R.D. Yedery, and C. Aranha. "Antimicrobial Peptides: Premises and Promises." *Journal of Antimicrobial Agents* 24, no 6 (December 2004): 536–47. http://www.ijaaonline.com/article/S0924-8579(04)00322-X/fulltext.

37 Bull, Matthew J., BSc, PhD, and Nigel T. Plummer, PhD. "Part 1: The Human Gut Microbiome in Health and Disease." *Integrative Medicine: A Clinician's Journal* 13, no 6 (Dec. 2014): 17–22. https://www.ncbi.nlm.nih. gov/pmc/articles/PMC4566439/.

38 "Allergy Facts and Figures." Asthma and Allergy Foundation of America. Accessed July 7, 2017. http://www.aafa.org/page/allergy-facts.aspx. "Allergies Statistics and Facts." *Healthline.* Accessed November 9, 2018. https://www.healthline.com/health/allergies/statistics#1. Guilleminault, Laurent, Evan J. Williams, Hayley A. Scott, et al. "Diet and Asthma: Is It

Time to Adapt Our Message?" *Nutrients* 9, no 11 (November 2017): 1227. https://www.ncbi.nlm.nih.gov/pmc/articles/PMC5707699/.

39   Ridlon, Jason M., Dae Joong Kang, Phillip B. Hylemon, et al. "Bile Acids and the Gut Microbiome." *Current Opinion in Gastroenterology* 30, no 3 (May 2014): 332–38. https://www.ncbi.nlm.nih.gov/pmc/articles/PMC4215539/#R28.

40   Boyer, James L. "Bile Formation and Secretion." *Comprehensive Physiology* 3, no 3 (July 2013): 1035–78. https://www.ncbi.nlm.nih.gov/pmc/articles/PMC4091928/. "Secretion of Bile and the Role of Bile Acids in Digestion." *Digestive System, Vivo Pathophysiology.* Accessed January 30, 2018. http://www.vivo.colostate.edu/hbooks/pathphys/digestion/liver/bile.html.

41   Hofmann, Alan F., and Lars Eckmann. "How Bile Acids Confer Gut Mucosal Protection Against Bacteria." *PNAS* 103, no 12 (March 21, 2006): 4333–34. https://www.ncbi.nlm.nih.gov/pmc/articles/PMC1450168/. Ridlon, 332–38.

42   Schmitz, G., and G. Müller. "Structure and Function of Lamellar Bodies, Lipid-Protein Complexes Involved in Storage and Secretion of Cellular Lipids." *Journal of Lipid Research* 32, no 10 (October 1991): 1539–70. https://www.ncbi.nlm.nih.gov/pubmed/1797938. Stremmel, W., R. Ehehalt, S. Staffer, et al. "Mucosal Protection by Phosphatidylcholine." *Digestive Diseases* 30, Suppl. 3 (2012): 85–91. https://www.karger.com/Article/Abstract/342729.

43   North Shore-Long Island Jewish Health System. "How the Immune System and Brain Communicate to Control Disease." *ScienceDaily,* July 22, 2008. https://www.sciencedaily.com/releases/2008/07/080721173748.htm.

44   Cryan, J.F. and T.G. Dinan. "Mind-altering Microorganisms: the Impact of the Gut Microbiota on Brain and Behaviour." *Nature Reviews. Neuroscience* 13, no 10 (October 2012): 701–12. https://www.ncbi.nlm.nih.gov/pubmed/22968153/.

45   Wang, Yan, and Lloyd H. Kasper. "The Role of Microbiome in Central Nervous System Disorders." *Brain, Behavior, and Immunity* 38 (May 2014): 1–12. https://www.ncbi.nlm.nih.gov/pmc/articles/PMC4062078/.

46   North Shore-Long Island Jewish Health System. "How the Immune System and Brain Communicate to Control Disease." *ScienceDaily,* July 22, 2008. https://www.sciencedaily.com/releases/2008/07/080721173748.htm.

47   Wang, S.Z., S. Li, X.Y. Xu, et al. "Effect of Slow Abdominal Breathing Combined with Biofeedback on Blood Pressure and Heart Rate Variability in Prehypertension." *Journal of Alternative and Complementary Medicine*

16, no 10 (October 2010): 1039–45. https://www.ncbi.nlm.nih.gov/pubmed/20954960.

48 Lehrer, Paul M., and Richard Gevirtz. "Heart Rate Variability Biofeedback: How and Why Does It Work?" *Frontiers in Psychology*, July 21, 2014. https://www.frontiersin.org/articles/10.3389/fpsyg.2014.00756/full.

49 Oaklander, Mandy and Robert Dantzer. "Cytokine, Sickness Behavior, and Depression." *Immunology and Allergy Clinics of North America* 29, no 2 (May 2009): 247–64. https://www.ncbi.nlm.nih.gov/pmc/articles/PMC2740752/

50 Becker, Robert O., and Gary Selden. *The Body Electric*. New York: William Morrow and Company, Inc., 1985.

51 Kobayashi, Masaki, Daisuke Kikuchi, and Hitoshi Okamura. "Imaging of Ultraweak Spontaneous Photon Emission from Human Body Displaying Diurnal Rhythm." *PLOS One*, July 16, 2009. http://journals.plos.org/plosone/article?id=10.1371/journal.pone.0006256.

52 Ibid.

53 Thaik, Cynthia M., MD. "Our Emotions Can Damage the Heart." *Psychology Today*, March 19, 2014. https://www.psychologytoday.com/blog/the-heart/201403/our-emotions-can-damage-the-heart-0.

54 Bhattacharya, Shaoni. "Brain Study Links Negative Emotions and Lowered Immunity." New Scientist, Sept. 2, 2003. https://www.newscientist.com/article/dn4116-brain-study-links-negative-emotions-and-lowered-immunity/.

55 Emoto, Masaru. *The Hidden Messages in Water*. Atria Books, 2001, p. 68.

56 Stellar, J.E., N. John-Henderson, C.L. Anderson, et al. "Positive Affect and Markers of Inflammation: Discrete Positive Emotions Predict Lower Levels of Inflammatory Cytokines." *Emotion* 15, no 2 (April 2015): 129–33. https://www.ncbi.nlm.nih.gov/pubmed/25603133. Castillo, Stephanie. "Awe-Inspiring Moments Lower Inflammation Marker Cytokines, Positively Impact Health." *MedicalDaily*, April 3, 2015. http://www.medicaldaily.com/awe-inspiring-moments-lower-inflammation-marker-cytokines-positively-impact-health-328092.

CHAPTER FOUR
How Disease Takes Hold: When the Seesaw Starts to Tip

57 Safe Drinking Water Act, Environmental Protection Agency. Accessed March 26, 2017. https://www.epa.gov/sdwa. Duhigg, Charles. "The Tap

Water Is Legal but May Be Unhealthy." *The New York Times*, December 16, 2009. http://www.nytimes.com/2009/12/17/us/17water.html.

58   Trautmann, Nancy M., Keith S. Porter, and Robert J. Wagenet. "Modern Agriculture: Its Effects on the Environment." Cornell University Cooperative Extension Pesticide Safety Education Program. Accessed March 26, 2017. http://psep.cce.cornell.edu/facts-slides-self/facts/mod-ag-grw85.aspx.

59   "National Primary Drinking Water Regulations." Environmental Protection Agency. Accessed March 26, 2017. https://www.epa.gov/ground-water-and-drinking-water/national-primary-drinking-water-regulations#Inorganic.

60   Duhigg, Charles. "The Tap Water Is Legal but May Be Unhealthy." *The New York Times*, December 16, 2009. http://www.nytimes.com/2009/12/17/us/17water.html.

61   Lambert, Craig. "The Way We Eat Now." *Harvard Magazine*, May–June, 2004. http://harvardmagazine.com/2004/05/the-way-we-eat-now.html.

62   Buttorff, Christine, Teague Ruder, and Melissa Bauman. "Multiple Chronic Conditions in the United States." Rand Corporation, 2017. https://www.rand.org/pubs/tools/TL221.html.

63   Samsel, Anthony and Stephanie Seneff. 9–46; Davis, D.R., M.D. Epp, and H.D. Riordan. "Changes in USDA Food Composition Data for 43 Garden Crops, 1950 to 1999." *Journal of the American College of Nutrition* 23, no 6 (December 2004): 669–82. https://www.ncbi.nlm.nih.gov/pubmed/15637215. "Dirt Poor: Have Fruits and Vegetables Become Less Nutritious?" *Scientific American.* Accessed February 4, 2018. https://www.scientificamerican.com/article/soil-depletion-and-nutrition-loss/.

64   Davis, D.R., M.D. Epp, and H.D. Riordan. "Changes in USDA Food Composition Data for 43 Garden Crops, 1950 to 1999." *Journal of the American College of Nutrition* 23, no 6 (December 2004): 669–82. https://www.ncbi.nlm.nih.gov/pubmed/15637215

65   "How Much Sugar Do You Eat? You May Be Surprised!" New Hampshire Department of Health and Human Services. Accessed February 4, 2018. https://www.dhhs.nh.gov/dphs/nhp/documents/sugar.pdf. Lenoir, Magalie, Fuschia Serre, Lauriane Cantin, et al. "Intense Sweetness Surpasses Cocaine Reward." *PLOS One* 2, no 8 (August 1, 2007): e698. https://www.ncbi.nlm.nih.gov/pmc/articles/PMC1931610/.

66   Steele, Eurídice Martínez, Larissa Galastri Baraldi, Maria Laura da Costa Louzada, et al. "Ultra-Processed Foods and Added Sugars in the US Diet:

Evidence from a Nationally Representative Cross-Sectional Study." *BMJ Open* 6, no 3 (January 1, 2016). http://bmjopen.bmj.com/content/6/3/e009892.

67 Yang, Qing. "Gain Weight by 'Going Diet?' Artificial Sweeteners and the Neurobiology of Sugar Cravings." *Yale Journal of Biology and Medicine* 83, no 2 (June 2010): 101–8. https://www.ncbi.nlm.nih.gov/pmc/articles/PMC2892765/. Conti, Lisa. "Artificial Sweeteners Confound the Brain; May Lead to Diet Disaster." *Scientific American*, June 1, 2008. https://www.scientificamerican.com/article/artificial-sweeteners-confound-the-brain/.

68 Schernhammer, Eva S., Kimberly A. Bertrand, and Brenda M. Birmann. "Consumption of Artificial Sweetener- and Sugar-Containing Soda and Risk of Lymphoma and Leukemia in Men and Women." *The American Journal of Clinical Nutrition* 96, no 6 (Dec. 2012): 1419–28. http://www.cspinet.org/new/pdf/aspartame%20Schernhammer%202012.pdf.

69 "Names of Ingredients That Contain Processed Free Glutamic Acid (MSG) *1." The Truth in Labeling Campaign. Accessed February 11, 2019. https://www.truthinlabeling.org/hiddensources.html.

70 Miller, Anna Medaris. "Should You Be Worried About Food Dyes?" *U.S. News*. Accessed October 8, 2017. https://health.usnews.com/wellness/articles/2016-03-17/should-you-be-worried-about-food-dyes.

71 Dunn, John T. "What's Happening to Our Iodine?" *The Journal of Clinical Endocrinology & Metabolism*, 83, no 10 (October 1, 1998): 3398–3400. https://academic.oup.com/jcem/article/83/10/3398/2865250.

72 Santarelli, Raphaëlle L., Fabrice Pierre, Denis E. Corpet. "Processed Meat and Colorectal Cancer: a Review of Epidemiology and Experimental Evidence." *Nutrition and Cancer* 60, no 2 (2008): 131–44. https://www.ncbi.nlm.nih.gov/pmc/articles/pmc2661797/.

73 Cressey, Daniel. "Widely Used Herbicide Linked to Cancer." *Nature*. March 24, 2015. https://www.nature.com/news/widely-used-herbicide-linked-to-cancer-1.17181. Gillam, Carey. "FDA Finds Monsanto's Weed Killer in US Honey." *Huffington Post*, September 15, 2016. http://www.huffingtonpost.com/carey-gillam/fda-finds-monsantos-weed_b_12008680.html. Honeycutt, Zen. "Monsanto's Glyphosate Found in California Wines, Even Wines Made with Organic Grapes." *EcoWatch*, March 27, 2016. https://www.ecowatch.com/monsantos-glyphosate-found-in-california-wines-even-wines-made-with-or-1882199552.html.

74 Type 2 Diabetes Statistics and Facts. *Healthline*. Accessed February 9, 2019.

https://www.healthline.com/health/type-2-diabetes/statistics#1.

75   "Statistics About Diabetes." American Diabetes Association. Accessed July
     1, 2017. http://www.diabetes.org/diabetes-basics/statistics/?loc=db-slabnav.

76   Goodman, Sara. "Tests Find More Than 200 Chemicals in Newborn
     Umbilical Cord Blood." *Scientific American*, December 2, 2009. https://www.
     scientificamerican.com/article/newborn-babies-chemicals-exposure-bpa/.

77   Urbina, Ian. "Think Those Chemicals Have Been Tested?" *The New York
     Times*, April 13, 2013. http://www.nytimes.com/2013/04/14/sunday-review/
     think-those-chemicals-have-been-tested.html.

78   Nordqvist, Christian. "What Is a Food Intolerance?" *Medical News Today*,
     December 20, 2017. https://www.medicalnewstoday.com/articles/263965.
     php. Giugliano D., A. Ceriello, and K. Esposito. "The Effects of Diet on
     Inflammation—Emphasis on the Metabolic Syndrome." *Journal of the
     American College of Cardiology* 48, no 4 (August 15, 2006): 677–85. https://
     www.ncbi.nlm.nih.gov/pubmed/16904534.

79   Celiac Disease Facts and Figures. The University of Chicago Medicine
     Celiac Disease Center. Accessed February 27, 2018. https://www.
     cureceliacdisease.org/wp-content/uploads/341_CDCFactSheets8_
     FactsFigures.pdf.

80   De Punder, Karin, and Leo Pruimboom. "The Dietary Intake of Wheat
     and Other Cereal Grains and Their Role in Inflammation." *Nutrients* 5,
     no 3 (March 2013): 771–87. https://www.ncbi.nlm.nih.gov/pmc/articles/
     PMC3705319/.

81   Ojetti V., G. Nucera, A. Migneco, et al. "High Prevalence of Celiac Disease in
     Patients with Lactose Intolerance." Digestion 71, no 2 (2005): 106–10. https://
     www.ncbi.nlm.nih.gov/pubmed/15775678. Fitterman, Lisa. "When Dairy
     Intolerance Joins Celiac Disease." Allergic Living, March 26, 2013. https://www.
     allergicliving.com/2013/03/26/when-dairy-intolerance-joins-celiac-disease/.

82   Malekinejad, Hassan, and Rezabakhsh, Aysa. "Hormones in Dairy Foods and
     Their Impact on Public Health–A Narrative Review Article." *Iranian Journal
     of Public Health* 44, no 6 (June 2015): 742–58. https://www.ncbi.nlm.nih.gov/
     pmc/articles/PMC4524299/.

83   Kiecolt-Glaser, Janice K., PhD. "Stress, Food, and Inflammation:
     Psychoneuroimmunology and Nutrition at the Cutting Edge." *Psychosomatic
     Medicine* 72, no 4 (May 2010): 365–69. https://www.ncbi.nlm.nih.gov/pmc/
     articles/PMC2868080/.

84 "Small Intestine." *InnerBody.Com.* Accessed February 6, 2018. http://www.
innerbody.com/image_digeov/dige10-new3.html.

85 Fasano, Alessio. "Zonulin, Regulation of Tight Junctions, and Autoimmune
Diseases." *Annals of the New York Academy of Sciences* 1258, no 1 (July
2012): 25–33. https://www.ncbi.nlm.nih.gov/pmc/articles/PMC3384703/.

86 Tchounwou, Paul B., Clement G. Yedjou, Anita K. Patlolla, et al. "Heavy
Metals Toxicity and the Environment." *Experientia. Supplementum.* no
101 (April 24, 2012): 133–64. https://www.ncbi.nlm.nih.gov/pmc/articles/
PMC4144270/.

87 Sherlach, Katy S., Alexander P. Gorka, Alexa Dantzler, et al. "Quantification
of Perchloroethylene Residues in Dry-Cleaned Fabrics." *Environmental
Toxicology and Chemistry* 30, no 11 (August 26, 2011): 2481–87. https://
setac.onlinelibrary.wiley.com/doi/epdf/10.1002/etc.665?referrer_
access_token=XZxcva4cI6-Wx092UqS4gE4keas67K9QMdWULT
WMo8NyWXN-0b1VrSCWUaOOCczpMb6v-RMDkFRKXVCZl_
eLjU8VXJrdHQi35NThA8hp1B7bkGtlbHTexZqOnT9BgYUg.
"Tetrachloroethylene (Perchloroethylene)." Environmental Protection
Agency. Accessed May 18, 2018. https://www.epa.gov/sites/production/
files/2016-09/documents/tetrachloroethylene.pdf.

88 Steinemann, Anne C. "Volatile Emissions from Common Consumer
Products." *Air Quality, Atmosphere & Health* 8, no 3 (June 2015): 273–81.
https://link.springer.com/article/10.1007/s11869-015-0327-6. Steinemann,
Anne C., Lisa G. Gallagher, and Amy L. Davis. "Chemical Emissions from
Residential Dryer Vents During Use of Fragranced Laundry Products." *Air
Quality, Atmosphere & Health* 6, no 1 (March 2013): 151–56. https://link.
springer.com/article/10.1007/s11869-011-0156-1.

89 Bottoni, P., S. Caroli, and A. Barra Caracciolo. "Pharmaceuticals as
Priority Water Contaminants." *Toxicology & Environmental Chemistry*
92, no 3 (March 12, 2010): 549–65. https://www.tandfonline.com/doi/
abs/10.1080/02772241003614320. Romo, Vanessa. "Traces of Opioids Found
in Seattle-Area Mussels." *NPR* (May 25, 2018). https://www.npr.org/sections/
thetwo-way/2018/05/25/614593382/traces-of-opioids-found-in-seattle-area-
mussels. Drugs in the Water. *Harvard Health Letter,* June 2011. https://www.
health.harvard.edu/newsletter_article/drugs-in-the-water.

90 Emoto, p. xxiii.

91 Mirza, Ambreen, Andrew King, and Claire Troakes. "Aluminum in

Brain Tissue in Familial Alzheimer's Disease." *Toxicology* 40 (March 2017): 30–36. https://www.sciencedirect.com/science/article/pii/S0946672X16303777.

92   "Mercury Can Jump Barrier That Keeps Toxins Out of Brain." *ScienceDaily*, September 9, 1999. https://www.sciencedaily.com/releases/1999/09/990909080318.htm. Yuan, Guiping, Hongke Lu, Zhongqiong Yin, et al. "Effects of Mixed Subchronic Lead Acetate and Cadmium Chloride on Bone Metabolism in Rats." *International Journal of Clinical and Experimental Medicine* 7, no 5 (2014): 1378–85. https://www.ncbi.nlm.nih.gov/pmc/articles/PMC4073760/.

93   "The Trouble with Ingredients in Sunscreens." *EWG's Guide to Sunscreens.* Accessed April 23, 2018. https://www.ewg.org/sunscreen/report/the-trouble-with-sunscreen-chemicals/#.Wt54UNPwbPA.

94   "Kohl, Kajal, Al-Kahal, Surma, Tiro, Tozali, or Kwalli: By Any Name, Beware of Lead Poisoning." US Food & Drug Administration. Accessed February 2, 2018. https://www.fda.gov/Cosmetics/ProductsIngredients/Products/ucm137250.htm. LaMotte, Sandee. "Claire's Pulls Children's Makeup Kits Over Asbestos Concerns." *CNN*, December 29, 2017. https://www.cnn.com/2017/12/29/health/claires-asbestos-child-makeup/index.html. Hepp, Nancy M. "Determination of Total Lead in 400 Lipsticks on the US Market Using a Validated Microwave-assisted Digestion, Inductively Coupled Plasma-mass Spectrometric Method." *Journal of the Society of Cosmetic Chemists* 63, no 3 (2012): 159–76. http://journal.scconline.org/abstracts/cc2012/cc063n03/p00159-p00176.html. "Limiting Lead in Lipsticks and Other Cosmetics." US Food & Drug Administration. Accessed February 2, 2018. https://www.fda.gov/Cosmetics/ProductsIngredients/Products/ucm137224.htm.

95   Raz, Amir. "Could Certain Frequencies of Electromagnetic Waves or Radiation Interfere with Brain Function?" *Scientific American.* Accessed October 8, 2017. https://www.scientificamerican.com/article/could-certain-frequencies/.

96   Koch, Holger M. and Antonia M. Calaft. "Human Body Burdens of Chemicals Used in Plastic Manufacture." *Philosophical Transactions of the Royal Society of London.* 364, no 1526 (July 27, 2009): 2063–78. https://www.ncbi.nlm.nih.gov/pmc/articles/pmc2873011/. Lloyd, Robin. "'Chemical Body Burden' Researchers and Advocates Raise Questions About Biomonitoring Studies and Hazards Regulations." *Scientific American.* February 20, 2011. https:// blogs.scientificamerican.com/observations/

chemical-body-burden-researchers-and-advocates-raise-questions-about-biomonitoring-studies-and-hazards-regulations/.

97 "31 Million Americans Skip Breakfast." *Huffington Post*, October 10, 2011. https://www.huffingtonpost.com/2011/10/11/31-million-americans-skip_n_1005076.html.

98 Cohen, Erica, Roger Bolus, Dinesh Khanna, et al. "GERD Symptoms in the General Population: Prevalence and Severity Versus Care-Seeking Patients." *Digestive Diseases and Sciences* 59, no 10 (October 2014): 2488–96. https://www.ncbi.nlm.nih.gov/pmc/articles/PMC4275099/. Pietrangelo, Ann. "GERD by the Numbers: Facts, Statistics & You." *Healthline*. March 2, 2015. https://www.healthline.com/health/gerd/facts-statistics-infographic#1. Gann, Carrie. "Reports of Frequent Heartburn Double, Study Says." *ABC News*. December 21, 2011. https://abcnews.go.com/Health/acid-reflux-rise-study-finds/story?id=15208938.

99 "Weight Loss Combined with Vitamin D Reduces Inflammation Linked to Cancer, Chronic Disease." Fred Hutchinson Cancer Research Center, June 24, 2015. https://www.fredhutch.org/en/news/releases/2015/06/weight-loss-plus-vitamin-d-reduces-inflammation.html.

100 Keylock, K. Todd, Victoria J. Vieira, Matthew A. Wallig, et al. "Exercise Accelerates Cutaneous Wound Healing and Decreases Wound Inflammation in Aged Mice." *American Journal of Physiology* 294, no 1 (January 1, 2008): R179–84. https://www.physiology.org/doi/10.1152/ajpregu.00177.2007. Hamer, Mark, PhD., Severine Sabia, PhD, G. David Batty, PhD, et al. "Physical Activity and Inflammatory Markers Over 10 Years Follow Up in Men and Women from the Whitehall II Cohort Study." *Circulation* 126, no 8 (August 21, 2012): 928–33. https://www.ncbi.nlm.nih.gov/pmc/articles/PMC3890998/.

101 "Poor Sleep Quality Increases Inflammation, Community Study Finds." Emory Woodruff Health Sciences Center, News Release, November 15, 2010. http://shared.web.emory.edu/whsc/news/releases/2010/11/poor-sleep-quality-increases-inflammation-study-finds.html.

102 Li, Xiaojing, Kristin M. Kolltveit, Leif Tronstad, et al. "Systemic Diseases Caused by Oral Infection." *Clinical Microbiology Reviews* 13, no 4 (October 2000): 547–58. https://www.ncbi.nlm.nih.gov/pmc/articles/PMC88948/. Liljestrand, J.M., P. Mantyla, S. Paju, et al. "Association of Endodontic Lesions with Coronary Artery Disease." *Journal of Dental Research* 95, no 12 (November 1, 2016). http://journals.sagepub.com/

doi/10.1177/0022034516660509.

CHAPTER FIVE
Balancing the Seesaw: What Keeps Us Well

103 Ignarro, L.J., M.L. Balestrieri, and C. Napoli. "Nutrition, Physical Activity and Cardiovascular Disease: An Update." *Cardiovascular Research* 73, no 2 (January 15, 2007): 326–40. https://www.ncbi.nlm.nih.gov/pubmed/16945357. Block, G., B. Patterson, and A. Subar. "Fruit, Vegetables, and Cancer Prevention: A Review of the Epidemiological Evidence." *Nutrition and Cancer* 18, no 1 (1992): 1–29. https://www.ncbi.nlm.nih.gov/pubmed/1408943.

104 Crinnion, W.J. "Organic Foods Contain Higher Levels of Certain Nutrients, Lower Levels of Pesticides, and May Provide Health Benefits for the Consumer." *Alternative Medicine Review* 15, no 1 (April 2010): 4–12. https://www.ncbi.nlm.nih.gov/pubmed/20359265.

105 Story, Erica N., Rachel E. Kopec, and Steven J. Schwartz. "An Update on the Health Effects of Tomato Lycopene." *Annual Review of Food Science and Technology* 1 (April 10, 2010): 189–210. https://www.annualreviews.org/doi/abs/10.1146/annurev.food.102308.124120?rfr_dat=cr_pub%3Dpubmed&url_ver=Z39.88-2003&rfr_id=ori%3Arid%3Acrossref.org&journalCode=food.

106 Panche, A.N., A.D. Diwan, and S.R. Chandra. "Flavonoids: An Overview," *Journal of Nutritional Science* 5 (December 2016): e47. https://www.ncbi.nlm.nih.gov/pmc/articles/PMC5465813/.

107 Konczak, Izabela and Wei Zhang. "Anthocyanins—More Than Nature's Colours," *Journal of Biomedicine and Biotechnology* 5 (December 1, 2004): 239–40. https://www.ncbi.nlm.nih.gov/pmc/articles/PMC1082903/.

108 Hebeisen, D.F., F. Hoeflin, H.P. Reusch, et al. "Increased Concentrations of Omega-3 Fatty Acids in Milk and Platelet Rich Plasma of Grass-Fed Cows." *International Journal for Vitamin and Nutrition Research* 63, no 3 (1993): 229–33. https://www.ncbi.nlm.nih.gov/pubmed/7905466.

109 Romo, Vanessa. "Traces of Opioids Found in Seattle-Area Mussels." NPR (May 25, 2018). https://www.npr.org/sections/thetwo-way/2018/05/25/614593382/traces-of-opioids-found-in-seattle-area-mussels.

110 "Plastic Bottles Release Potentially Harmful Chemicals (Bisphenol A) After Contact with Hot Liquids." *ScienceDaily* (February 4, 2008). https://www.

sciencedaily.com/releases/2008/01/080130092108.htm.

111 Sundar, Shyam and Jaya Chakravarty. "Antimony Toxicity." *International Journal of Environmental Research and Public Health* 7, no 12 (December 2010): 4267–77. https://www.ncbi.nlm.nih.gov/pmc/articles/PMC3037053/. Fan, Ying-Ying, Jian-Lun Zheng, Jing-Hau Ren, et al. "Effects of Storage Temperature and Duration on Release of Antimony and Bisphenol A from Polyethylene Terephthalate Drinking Water Bottles of China." Environmental Pollution 192 (September 2014): 113–20. https://www.sciencedirect.com/science/article/pii/S0269749114002000?via%3Dihub.

112 Johnson, Mats, Sven Östlund, Gunnar Fransson, et al. "Omega-3/Omega-6 Fatty Acids for Attention Deficit Hyperactivity Disorder: A Randomized Placebo-Controlled Trial in Children and Adolescents." *Journal of Attention Disorders* 12, no 5 (March 1, 2009): 394–401. http://journals.sagepub.com/doi/abs/10.1177/1087054708316261. Su, Kuan-Pin, Yutaka Matsuoka, and Chi-Un Pae. "Omega-3 Polyunsaturated Fatty Acids in Prevention of Mood and Anxiety Disorders." *Clinical Psychopharmacology and Neuroscience* 13, no 2 (August 2015): 129–37. https://www.ncbi.nlm.nih.gov/pmc/articles/PMC4540034/. Tsaluchidu, Sofia, Massimo Cocchi, and Lucio Tonello. "Fatty Acids and Oxidative Stress in Psychiatric Disorders." *BMC Psychiatry* 8, Supplement 1 (April 17, 2008): S5. https://bmcpsychiatry.biomedcentral.com/articles/10.1186/1471-244X-8-S1-S5. Freeman, M.P., J.R. Hibbeln, K.L. Wisner, et al. "Omega-3 Fatty acids: Evidence Basis for Treatment and Future Research in Psychiatry." *The Journal of Clinical Psychiatry* 67, no 2 (December 2006): 1954–67. https://www.ncbi.nlm.nih.gov/pubmed/17194275. Yehuda, S., S. Rabinovitz, and D.I. Mostofsky. "Essential Fatty Acids Are Mediators of Brain Biochemistry and Cognitive Functions." *Journal of Neuroscience Research* 56, no 6 (June 15, 1999): 565–70. https://www.ncbi.nlm.nih.gov/pubmed/10374811.

113 "How to Optimize Your Omega-6 to Omega-3 Ratio." *Healthline.* Accessed February 9, 2018. https://www.healthline.com/nutrition/optimize-omega-6-omega-3-ratio.

114 Daley, Cynthia A., Amber Abbott, Patrick Doyle, et al. "A Review of Fatty Acid Profiles and Antioxidant Content in Grass-Fed and Grain-Fed Beef." *Nutrition Journal* 9 (March 10, 2010): 10. https://nutritionj.biomedcentral.com/articles/10.1186/1475-2891-9-10.

115 Rodriguez, Nancy R. "Introduction to Protein Summit 2.0: Continued Exploration of the Impact of High-Quality Protein on Optimal Health." *The*

American Journal of Clinical Nutrition 101, no 6 (June 1, 2015): 1317s–19s. https://academic.oup.com/ajcn/article/101/6/1317S/4564491.

116 "13 Ways to a Healthy Liver." October 2013, American Liver Foundation. http://www.liverfoundation.org/education/liverlowdown/ll1013/13ways/.

117 Finley, Bruce. "Deciduous Trees Have Decidedly Beneficial Impact on Air Pollution." The Denver Post, October 21, 2000 (updated May 5, 2016). http://www.denverpost.com/2010/10/21deciduous-trees-have-decidedly-beneficial-impact-on-air-pollution/.

118 Sears, Margaret E., Kathleen J. Kerr, and Riina I. Bray. "Arsenic, Cadmium, Lead, and Mercury in Sweat: A Systematic Review." *Journal of Environmental and Public Health*, 2012. https://www.hindawi.com/journals/jeph/2012/184745/.

119 Young, Simon N. "Folate and Depression—a Neglected Problem." *Journal of Psychiatry & Neuroscience* 32, no 2 (March 2007): 80–82. https://www.ncbi.nlm.nih.gov/pmc/articles/PMC1810582/.

120 "Vitamin B$_6$." Michigan Medicine, University of Michigan. Accessed February 28, 2018. http://www.uofmhealth.org/health-library/hn-2928009.

121 Coppen, A., and C. Bolander-Gouaille. "Treatment of Depression: Time to Consider Folic Acid and Vitamin B$_{12}$." *Journal of Psychopharmacology* 19, no 1 (January 2005): 59–65. https://www.ncbi.nlm.nih.gov/pubmed/15671130. Briani, C., C. Dalla Torre, V. Citton, et al. "Cobalamin Deficiency: Clinical Picture and Radiological Findings." *Nutrients* 5, no 11 (November 15, 2013): 4521–39. https://www.ncbi.nlm.nih.gov/pubmed/24248213.

122 "MTHFR Gene." *Genetics Home Reference.* US National Library of Medicine. Accessed April 6, 2018. https://ghr.nlm.nih.gov/gene/MTHFR. "MTHFR Gene Variant." *Genetic and Rare Diseases Information Center.* NIH National Center for Advancing Translational Sciences. Accessed April 6, 2018. https://rarediseases.info.nih.gov/diseases/10953/mthfr-gene-mutation.

123 Vogel, Lauren. "Hand Sanitizers May Increase Norovirus Risk." *Canadian Medical Association Journal* 183, no 12 (September 6, 2001): E799–E800. https://www.ncbi.nlm.nih.gov/pmc/articles/PMC3168661/. Stoker, T.E., E. K. Gibson, and L.M. Zorrilla. "Triclosan Exposure Modulates Estrogen-Dependent Responses in the Female Wistar Rat." *Toxicological Sciences* 117, no 1 (September 2010): 45–53. https://www.ncbi.nlm.nih.gov/pubmed/20562219.

ABOUT THE AUTHOR

Kristine L. Gedroic, MD, is the Medical Director of The Gedroic Medical Institute, in Morristown, New Jersey. Dr. Gedroic has helped patients with nearly every chronic condition, including autoimmune disease, neurological conditions, chronic fatigue syndrome, ADHD, depression, and more. She graduated from Harvard University with a degree in biochemical sciences and from Thomas Jefferson University Medical School. Dr. Gedroic is a fellow of the American Boards of Family Medicine and Integrative Medicine and is Clinical Associate Professor in the Department of Medicine at Rutgers New Jersey Medical School. She lives in New Jersey with her family.